# Relentless

# Relentless

## Walking Against All Odds

Josh Wood

Angeleah Anton & Kay Ledson

First Published in Canada 2013 by Influence Publishing

Book Design: Marla Thompson
Typesetting: Greg Salisbury
Photographer: Nick Dale Photography

DISCLAIMER: This book has been created to inform individuals with an interest in taking back control of their own health. It is not intended in any way to replace other professional health care or mental health advice, but to support it. Readers of this publication agree that neither Josh Wood nor his publisher will be held responsible or liable for damages that may be alleged or resulting, directly, or indirectly, from their use of this publication. All external links are provided as a resource only and are not guaranteed to remain active for any length of time. Neither the publisher nor the author can be held accountable for the information provided by, or actions resulting from accessing these resources. All opinions in this book are those of the author.

I dedicate this book in the loving memory of my amazing mates and grandma who passed. You will never be forgotten nor will your legacy ever fade away. The love, knowledge, and strength you all gave me in your own way will forever sit heavy in my heart, and I promise to better my life every day in honour of what I have learned from each and all of you, until we meet again—

My bright stars in the sky and my guides through my life—Grandma Dottie, Judd Greedy, Bronte Holland, Matty McMillan, and Heath Gilmore.

I also dedicate this book to those who will never stop fighting for their dreams and goals. To those who are struck down by not just a spinal cord injury, but also illness, breakups, losses, or to those who just need a boost of motivation. Hopefully by me telling my story, I can at least help one person with whatever their struggle may be, big or small.

# Testimonials

## Gus Smarrini

### Practice Development Manager – MLC Australia

*"Josh Wood is an inspiration to everyone who is fortunate enough to hear his story of when apparent irrevocable tragedy meets unparalleled will and determination. He is a passionate, humble, yet entertaining young man whose message will leave you, your clients, and/or your staff with invaluable insight into what can be achieved when the human spirit refuses to surrender. I strongly recommend Josh as your keynote speaker at your next client function or team-building program. "*

## Robbie Maddison

### Multi-time World Record Holder, XGames Medalist, James Bond Stunt Double

*"A moving account of tragedy striking and an up-and-coming star destined for extreme glory. Positive energy and his mother's love starts Josh on his way to rewrite the medical journals. His will to live and mind-over-matter approach is truly inspiring."*

## Kathleen Ayris

### Project Manager Corporate Business Events MLC Melbourne, Australia

*"Josh delivered the closing presentation at our conference earlier this year. He received a standing ovation and left our audience inspired by his determination to overcome and repair his injuries to the best of his ability, against the prognosis of professionals."*

*The best thing about hearing someone tell their own story is that it doesn't have to be perfect! It was not over-rehearsed or too polished; it was real, believable, and powerful.*

*Josh has a real ability to connect with people at all levels and through his story telling he openly welcomes people into his world and his experiences. Josh's story touches on many themes and genres: motivational, inspirational, power of positive thinking, overcoming the impossible, beating the odds, insuring your children for the worst, the importance of insurance, and more! Josh's presentation received an average rating of 'outstanding' at our conference."*

# Acknowledgements

To the people I would like to thank for being there when my family and I needed you the most; you gave us support, motivation, and of course, love.

My family, family friends, and recovery team:

My mum Kay, my wife Amelia, our furry children Montana and Thor, aunties Susie and Wendy, Grandma Dottie, Gary Ledson and family, the in-laws Malcolm, Jude, Laura, and Thomas Allen, Asri, my dad Garry, his wife Chris, step-brother Andrew and his family, step-sister Karen and her family, cousins Mark and Ivy, Simon and Jennifer Floreani and the Vitality Middle Park team, Paula, Isabel, Bing, Jenny and James the acupuncturists, Dana and John Goyak, Dr. Graeme Baro, Uschi Schneider, Doug, Jackie, Bryony and the Cole Family, Marie Bermingham, the Morger family in Switzerland, the O'Malley family in Ireland, and Julie Bennett.

My mates:

Chris Bateup and family, Daniel Schulz and family, Paul De Bruyn and family, Luke ("Dingo") Trembath and family, Mark and James Peschel and family, Luke ("Lukey Luke") Follacchio and family, the Hobbo guys and girls, Thomas Laslo and family, Zayne Stoner, Boz and Alex Gurmesevic, Jade Hunt, Gavin Walker and family, Robbie Maddison and family, Josh Cachia and family, Shaun, Jane Brunton and family, Adam Smith, Todd, Tyson and Armani Stanley, Jason Shealsey, Mitch Vipond & family, Dwayne Curran and family, Dax, Jamie, Barb and the ASN Erina Team, Michele ("Miss Handgrenade") Phyman, Richard ("Dick"), Kristy, Demi, Kruse Lunt, Karl McCafferty and family, Matt Piva and Skullcandy family, Braden and Mario at New Era, Trigger Gumm and family, Graham, Holly Eves, Dominic and Jess Gasser and family, Hayden, and Sarah Graham.

My supporters and trainers:

Project Walk trainers, Tommy and the Fitlife Gym, Jason Sheppard, Jack and the Sweat Gym, Colin and Rosie McMillan, Ian and Andrew Lamerton and family, Sue, Brendan and Grady Holland, Julie and Rob Greedy and family, Tracey and Greg McDonald and family, Jeff, Nick Dale, Barney and Kate Miller, Marie Dillon, Tracy Osterfield, Lesli and Curt, Donna J. Ledson Family in Sonoma, everyone involved in the "Help Woody Ditch the Stick" fundraiser who donated items and funds, and The MLC Risk Life Retreat Team 2012.

And Nick Dale Photography, for making my vision a reality with his amazing photography skills.

Each and every one of you have played some sort of role in my life, my recovery, and most importantly, you all believed in me. Your love, care, and encouragement have given me a new lease on life, that in those early scary days I never thought was imaginable. You all keep me striving to achieve more and I can never thank you enough.

# Table of Contents

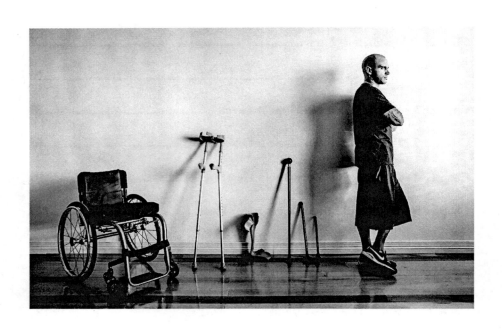

# Foreword

*"Challenges are what make life interesting and overcoming them is what makes life meaningful."*
**Joshua J. Marine**

"Josh Wood is a unique gift to my world. I used to think of him as a crazy young fool with a deep desire to hurt himself and his loved ones in the process. In the years before he burst his spinal column I thought I had seen him injure himself badly and then rise out of the ashes more than enough times. I am very happy Josh has now set down his story. It's one that cries out to be told—and not just because he is a classified quadriplegic who walks, but more for the nature of his recovery from a severe spinal cord injury in 2000.

Josh Wood is a challenge for us health professionals because he is guided by innate intelligence before authority and his results are like a stick in the eye for those who think they know the answers to the healing capacity of the human body.

You will get everything from Josh to bringing more of himself to the world through this book because we all need to believe more in possibility and to make our lives more meaningful. If you connect with him, then please take this story to those in need of meaning. Millions of people are suffering with spinal injury, neurological disease, brain dysfunction, ABI, and strokes, and they need hope.

Some of us find it hard to get out of bed and get to work on time because we are bored, but Josh Wood, in 'Relentless: Walking against all odds' shows us that there is meaning in that challenge of simply getting the body switched on and out of bed.

Josh Wood was easy to judge, and still is, until you read what he has done to pursue a dream with courage, commitment, dedication, perseverance, sacrifice, and then a few more injections of courage. His story, like those of so many other extraordinary athletes, is to a large degree about triumph over adversity, because he is the sort of person he is, it is also candid, funny and refreshingly honest.

Josh is an authentic next generation leader because he does not tell you to 'do' anything but 'shows' us all by being authentic. 'Relentless: Walking against all odds' shocks me as a professional and a parent; more importantly, it tugs on the heart and bellows loudly to the hard heads of my adolescent sons. His recovery story guides us all in mastering our fear of the future and whether we can be a success in our life.

Josh Wood has shown me that one persons version of impossible can be my version of possible."

**Dr. Simon Floreani, chiropractor and servant to the healing process.**

# Prologue

I was one of those hyper active kids who never sat still. Still to this day, my mum, Kay Ledson, takes every opportunity to remind me that even from the very beginning of her pregnancy carrying me, I constantly moved about.

For my first birthday, my grandparents, Peter and Dottie, presented me with a mini version BMX bike with training wheels. Mum said the training wheels lasted about an hour before I ripped them off and were never to be seen again. That was typical of me, riding a bike—minus the training wheels—before I could even walk properly.

I was barely a year old and I had no fear riding the BMX up and down the hallway tearing up the inside of our house. When I was done racing around all the furniture, I took the adventure outside and rode flat out on the pavement that wrapped around the house.

At age two, I got my first set of skis. They were a mini version of adult skis and no one could get me off them. Snow and snow sports had come into my life and this was just the beginning of my extreme sports experiences.

My dad, Garry Wood, took my enthusiasm of riding my BMX to a whole new level when he introduced motorbikes into my life. Dad had a bike of his own and I was his "little man" pillion passenger dressed up in my motorbike gear to match his. I took to bikes so well that I was soon given a motorbike of my own. Dad and I built a racetrack out the back of our property and I would ride my bike around for hours until it would run out of petrol and I would just fill up the tank from the number of jerry cans Dad had sitting around the yard, and I'd be off again, racing around the track for another couple more hours.

I was six years of age then, and showing all the signs that the course of my life was pretty well set to continue in these adrenaline rush sports and both my parents knew it.

The stunt man in me showed up when my parents bought a hobby farm in Mansfield when I turned seven. Two years after the purchase they built a family home for the three of us to live in and that's when my need for speed really took off. I had the perfect setting to hone my motorbike skills. While my parents worked on the house, I raced around on my purpose-built motorbike track. There was only rule: everyone had to ride in the same direction. That rule still didn't stop all the collisions, accidents, banged heads, broken toes, and other injuries I sustained.

My destiny appeared when I was 12 years of age—snowboarding. That was it as far as I was concerned; I found something that made me feel alive and I was really good at it. Yes I was good at BMX and motor cross and I could have just as easily continued on with those sports and further developed my skill and level of competition but snowboarding took me to a whole new level of passion for being out on the snow. I was definitely hooked and there was no stopping me.

When I was 15 years of age, I was lucky enough to go on a student exchange program to Switzerland. I stayed with the Morger Family in Schanis, south east of Zurich. They had three sons who were around the same age as me and their parents were really supportive of my growing passion for being on the snow.

While I was in Switzerland, I became friends with a group of local snowboarders. These guys were some of the best I had ever ridden and jumped with. Patrick and Broder were my two closest friends and the ones I rode with the most. I spent every spare moment I could on the snow with them. They snowboarded and built jumps at levels that I had never ridden or jumped at before and the terrain was beyond anything I had ever seen. I knew then I just wanted to live my life travelling, snow-boarding, and having adventures like these.

I came back to Melbourne after being in Switzerland for just under four months and put into practice everything I learned over in Europe. I did some pretty big jumps in Switzerland and I wanted to continue doing the same back here, so I started doing a lot of the jumps Kirsty Marshall used to do, which were the aerial ones. Aerial jumps propel the snowboarder straight up into the air, so when they come off the jump, they pretty much go straight up and then they come straight back down. For a young snowboarder, that's how I learned—I started snowboarding at such a young age and the sport of snowboarding was so young itself that they didn't have proper big snowboard jumps back then. So I used to practice on the big jumps that were used for competitions and that's what led me onto the competition circuits.

It wasn't long before I turned 18 years of age and snowboarding still held my attention more than my other choices of extreme sports of motor cross racing and BMX racing. I had built up a presence on the snowboarding circuit over the years and I was now a member of Team Buller. I had developed a determined competitive streak, so I started competing at Mount Buller and Thredbo. Those competitions added so many new experiences and elements to my life; I thought I was invincible and had a new confidence now that helped me to achieve more of the things I wanted in my life and all this just kept adding to the overall experiences I had snowboarding at some of the best snow resorts an 18-year-old could wish for, from the Victorian and New South Wales snow resorts to the Swiss Alps. Sure, there was always the risk of a jump turning pear-shaped, so before each one, I would run through a mental picture in my mind of the jump I was about to make and I would always picture myself landing, or at least over-jumping and not landing short. Not for a minute did I think my invincible theory was about to be tested in the most intense way.

The date of Sunday, 25 June 2000, became an equally important date in my life as my actual birthday of Friday, 13 November 1981. I feel like I have two "birth" dates because at 3:30 p.m. on 25 June 2000, on the snowfields at an alpine resort in Victoria, Australia, I had an experience that took away the life that I had known for the past 18 years and replaced it with something very different. In a split second, the course of my life had been permanently changed and I could never have imagined what was ahead of me and what I was going to go through.

I knew the minute my body hit the asphalt road I had broken my neck and I was in a shitload of trouble. There is something remarkable about the human body and how it immediately responds and switches into a kind of shutdown action to protect itself from further trauma. As much as I was relieved to be off the side of the mountain and on that rescue helicopter as it flew me to a major Melbourne trauma hospital, my mind was racing with all kinds of thoughts: what the doctors were going to tell me when I arrived and they had examined me, how my parents and family were going to react to any devastating news, and my poor mates that were still up at the mountain not knowing if they were ever going to see me again.

I had been in the hospital for three days when the doctors delivered the news that I was now a quadriplegic. It was fair to say my first reaction to that news wasn't a good one. At 18 years of age and be told I would most likely never get out of bed, not walk, not be able to do anything unassisted for any of the daily routines an able-bodied person does was like giving me a death sentence and right in that moment, I preferred death. I probably should have died on the asphalt road at the alpine resort.

My mum wasn't having any of that "me wanting to die." She said if I didn't die when I hit the road and broke my neck, then that was evidence enough that I wasn't meant to go that way at that moment and I had made a decision then to live and that's what I going to do—live!

Mum and I worked out a recovery plan. It involved surrounding ourselves with alternative and less-than-mainstream practitioners; there was not going to be anything conventional about me putting my broken body back together. I was going to walk out of the rehabilitation centre and I was going to have the support of my family and friends and this new committed group of healers to help me achieve it. And I did!

I was someone with a medically diagnosed spinal cord injury who was left with only 5 percent functional spinal cord, labeled a quadriplegic, and yet there I was walking out of the rehab centre some 18 weeks later after my accident and just days before my nineteenth birthday.

Has it all been smooth sailing since I walked out of rehab? Not in the slightest. My road to recovery hasn't been a smooth one; I have struggled with my demons on a daily basis since the accident and I still do today to some extent, but I don't give up. Giving up just isn't an option or a choice. And that's what makes the difference—never give up! Developing a mentoring program for other spinal cord injury patients, speaking to them and their families and giving them the encouragement to rebuild their lives, and pushing the boundaries and be relentless to achieve recovery results just like I did are some of the things that keep my purpose for what I am here to do.

Through the belief, the love, and the support of my beautiful wife, parents, family, friends, and the incredible group of healers and practitioners I placed in my life, I keep going and keep getting me out there to inform people about spinal cord injury. Education, information, steadfast belief, and visualization are the most powerful healing tools one has when dealing with accident, illness, or other life-changing events. Spinal cord injury doesn't mean your life is over; it means your life is different.

*"In life, we try so hard to get things we don't have, but we never sit back to appreciate what we do have. Having a spinal cord injury, all I want is to have my life back to where it was! So celebrate what you have; you never know when you could lose it all."*
**Josh Wood, 2012**

# Chapter 1

# Destined to Jump

## You never know what the next day will bring.

I remember the exact moment my body hit the asphalt road. I hit it that damn hard and the sounds on impact were so loud that everyone standing close to me and around the jump must have heard them.

The sound of the back of my neck and the bottom part of my helmet as they smashed onto the road surface.

The sound of my chin as it hit my chest and the initial crack as my neck broke.

The sound of my knees as they hit my ears.

The screaming noise of the metal edges of my snowboard as it came in contact with the asphalt road.

The sound of my body springing back in the opposite direction as it forced my head to slam backwards in between my shoulder blades.

And then, I heard a sound that dominated all the others—it was the most disturbing sound of all—the sound that my neck made as it snapped. It was like an explosion just went off in my neck. Hearing that sound gave me a sheer terror like nothing else I had ever experienced before.

I thought, *Fuck, that's not good… What have I just done?*

Considering the violence of the crash, which had me bouncing back-wards off the road, I actually managed to stop quite quickly. I finished up on the side of the road on the edge of the snow and lay on the left side of my body all twisted up with my left arm trapped underneath my back. My legs were all twisted in the other direction and my butt was flat on the ground—the same as my heels because I was still strapped onto my board. The position of my body was so contorted that I must have looked like a pretzel—a rounded mesh of body, helmet, armour, and snowboard, lying on the side of the road on the edge of the snow.

I couldn't believe I was fully conscious and alive. I probably should have been dead after my neck snapped like that on impact. I might have just cheated death, but that was nothing compared to the hell I experienced after this brutal crash.

I heard my mates run down the road and others shuffled through the snow just as fast as them. The sound of their snow boots pounded on the road became louder and louder as they came closer to where I lay.

Daniel was screaming out my name, "Josh... Josh!" It was so loud that it echoed all the way **down the hill.**

I only had a few seconds of time before the boys reached me. It felt much longer because my mind was running a frame-by-frame picture show in graphic detail, over and over again, of what just happened to me. My neck was broken, my body was twisted, my left arm was trapped underneath my back, and I didn't know what damage my legs were in. All I knew was that my legs were twisted in the opposite direction to my body.

And then the reality hit me that I just changed the course of my life in a split second.

I lay there thinking, *What the fuck have I just done? I've completely ruined my entire life over a jump...*

I was up at the local ski resort for two weeks in an apartment on the mountain. My mates Daniel Shultz, Luke "Dingo" Trembath, Chris Bateup, Simon O'Keefe, and some other friends of ours also travelled up the mountain and were staying around the hill in accommodation. Every day we randomly selected the activities that we were going to do that day and we mixed them up a bit.

Snowboarding was always a priority activity for us; as well, we built our own jumps and did multiple runs down them, which improved our boarding techniques. We were just enjoying life being young and free. It was another world for us when we were on the snow. We also liked to swim in the heated pools at the various hotels or hang out at the main pub located right in the heart of the village. It was the most popular pub on the mountain and our favourite place to unwind after a full day of boarding and being out on the snow.

The day of my accident started out just like any other day on the mountain. I got up around 7:00 a.m. and ate, dressed myself, and I thought I would spend my day working on my snowboard techniques. The best way to hone my skill was to test it on a jump. I needed a jump to practice on.

I thought, *Well, there are enough of the boys up here; they can help me build my own jump.*

I mentioned it to the boys that were in the apartment with me and they thought it was a cool idea, so right after breakfast, we started the search for the right spot to build the jump.

We picked up our snowboards and shovels and headed off to the main traffic run of the mountain that overlooks the mountain village. We rode on our snowboards down to the bottom of the main street run to the pub and caught up with a few of the boys who were getting ready to head out and make a jump of their own.

We sat and talked about possible sites to build my jump. My preference was to build one across the cat-track where the Kässbohrers and other snow machinery have access to the mountain. This was a mini road that allows snow machinery and tractors access the different locations of the mountain safely. The boys didn't like this location. They said it wasn't suitable because the snow coverage down there wasn't good enough. They suggested that we could find a better spot for the jump on the other side of the hill, the North side, which had a lot more snow coverage.

I was familiar with that area of the mountain and thought it was worth a look. The boys were keen to check it out, so we headed off in that direction and walked up the road to where the new access road was built. This part of the road on the mountain was fairly new. It was built and asphalted two years prior and I saw the area alongside it that appeared to have quite good snow coverage. We walked along a couple more sections of the road and sighted some possible spots that could work. Parts of the road were really high and had a big gap, which gave the potential for a wide, high jump.

My first thought was, *It would be pretty cool to jump this road because everyone's talked about it but no one's actually done it yet because the road is so new.*

After walking a bit further along the road, we came to an area I thought looked good. I could see just before the road turned to the left there was a part of it that came back around on itself, which formed a U-turn, and then it went back up the hill. That particular section had a very good coverage of snow on the down ramp and I felt the run-in would be long enough for me to get enough speed to go at it.

I believed the combination of the long run-in and the long slope down would give me enough speed and distance coming off the lip of the ramp, to drop into the lower slope, float over the asphalt road, and land safely on the snow. Speed and distance were obviously going to be the crucial factors in either the success or failure of me making this jump, so I had to get them exactly right and plan and design this jump accurately.

Safety was the next thing to sort out, so I started going through my checklist.

First, I always checked was the landing: I tested how deep it was, how compacted the snow was, the quality of the snow, and if it was safe to land on.

Secondly, I questioned was whether there would be enough coverage if I drifted to the left or the right of the jump.

Thirdly, I looked closely at the down ramp and made sure there were no obstructions, which means no rocks, no boulders, no holes, no hills, or anything like that because it had to be totally clear.

The fourth area to focus on was the run-in.

I went through my checklist again, exactly the same, for the landing. I had to figure out if I had enough distance from where I start to where the jump has to be built to get maximum speed. My speed and distance determine everything.

I was satisfied with the area and that particular spot, everything on my checklist was done, and the landing and run-in were all clear and looked good. All that was left to do was to figure out the exact spot to build the ramp and what sort of ramp we were going to build.

I had to consider the angle and the degree of the jump. Was it going to be a really high pitch or did it need to be more flat? Was it going to be long or short? All I knew at that stage was that it needed to totally clear the road so I could safely reach far enough into the snow on the other side.

I felt the best spot to place the ramp was approximately 16 feet from the road edge on the high side. Using the steeper area of the slope would easily give me a faster and smoother run down onto the jump and a greater speed floating off the ramp so I would be able to clear the road. I didn't think it needed to be a very high pitch jump because I was going to come in from an angle where I jump downwards. It didn't have to be a *booter* because that would boot me up into the air. It needed to be more of a *floater* because I needed to float across in a straighter line over to the other side. I knew then that the kind of ramp I needed to build had to be a six-foot floater.

I grouped the boys together who were there with me—Daniel, Dingo, Simon, and a few others—we needed to get moving and build the jump because we had taken too much time already just choosing the right spot. We started smoothing out the run-up and began to dig up snow from the surrounding area. We kept piling the snow to create the ramp height I needed, and we had created some really good height.

The boys came and went as we worked through the different stages of the build. Some went off and did a bit of snowboarding or had lunch and then came back to pack some more snow. At times, there was only Dingo and myself building up the ramp; we stopped to take photos at different stages and made sure it looked good.

Word had spread around the resort that we were building a jump over the road and within an hour, people came down to have a look at what was going on. By then, the ramp was built up really well so I decided it was time to test it. We grabbed a bunch of the snowboards and stacked them on top of each other to make a wall and rolled the snow into balls by stacking and rolling one layer on top of another. We didn't have a hell of a lot of snow around it by then, so we just used what we had, which was luckily enough.

We kept chipping away and built it higher and higher. When each section was completed, I practiced my run down the ramp several times. I glided down the ramp and slowed my speed down because I didn't want to come at it as if I was going to jump. I only needed enough speed to get an idea of what the ramp surface felt like under my board in case I needed to make any adjustments. At the same time, I pushed the snow, which made it as compact as possible, and then I just pulled off at the last minute and turned left or right just before the end. It was a really good way of flattening the snow out and getting rid of all the lumps.

I always did several practice runs like that because when I do the first run, it shows up spots that I didn't see or might have missed in the building stage. There could be a hole, or the snow has softened in one place, or people have walked across it so I have to make sure that everything is fixed up before I do the actual jump.

Every time we made an adjustment, I tested it with a couple more practice runs. I even got two of the boys to go down it to make sure the snow was as flat as possible. I did a few more practice runs and completed several more checks of the jump just to be sure. I even got Dingo and one of the other boys to practice a manoeuvre to get my speed up onto the ramp. It was like a slingshot action where the boys stood on either side of me, held my hands, and then ran forward as they dragged me along the snow. They then slingshot me so I had that quick injection of speed first up. We did it a few more times and it worked well. As an extra precaution, I salted the jump and run-in. Adding salt lowers the freezing point of water and melts the snow. When it refreezes, it hardens, which makes the jump more stable and the icy surface helps the jump to last longer. It could easily last the whole day in that hardened condition.

At this point, I stood back and had a really good look at the finished ramp and run-in. I was happy with what we built. I thought the jump looked good and we all did a great job with the whole process of building and the preparation of it. We put so much time into getting the right height and the overall design to look good. Now it was done and ready for me to suit up and do the jump.

I grabbed my gear and my board and sat down for a second to put some race wax on the underside of my snowboard. A waxed board is easier to control and glides better. It also helps to increase your speed, and speed was the most important thing I needed to have right when I hit the ramp so I could get the height and length to make the jump safely. The time was after 3 p.m. when I started pulling on my snowboard gear for the jump. I put on my armour, which was shaped like a turtle shell.

It covered my back and came up to the base of the back of my neck. My hoodie went over the armour and I zipped it up, and then I put my helmet on.

I was ready.

I spent the last bit of time reviewing the line I needed to take and the angle I was going to approach from. Daniel and Dingo were standing next to me.

Dingo said, "Dude, you don't have to do this, it's pretty crazy."

Daniel said, "Are you sure you really want to do this Josh? This jump is pretty stupid. It's big and you don't have to do it. There's no pressure to do anything."

I said to both of them, "Nah, it's alright."

I didn't think anything was going to go wrong.

I was at an age where I thought I was invincible and I wanted to prove to myself that I was capable of doing this jump. I had done hundreds of jumps over the seven-year period I had been snowboarding. While living in Europe, I did a 120-foot long jump in Switzerland, so I had no concerns about distance with this jump. In fact, this jump was actually shorter—the danger element was the asphalt road, which put me more at risk if I fell short and didn't clear it.

I had to give 100 percent commitment to this jump. There was no room for error. I checked it over one last time and then I turned around and started walking up the hill to the top of the slope. In those few short moments when I walked up the hill towards the jump, neither my mates nor I had any idea that it would be my last time to walk normally. We were all unaware how radically my life was about to change in those next few minutes.

When I reached the top, I looked down in front of me at the run-in onto the ramp and all the way down the jump, over the lower part of the road to the landing. Focusing on the spot where the landing was positioned was the most important part for me. Before every jump I did, I always visualized myself landing.

I could see Daniel and Simon standing on the road at the end to the left of the jump. We also arranged for a couple of the boys to watch the road to stop any traffic that came in front of the jumping area.

It was 3:30 p.m. and time to jump!

I had Dingo and one of the other boys stand on either side of me and they grabbed my hands.

Again, Dingo said, "Josh are you really 100 percent sure you want to do this?"

I said, "Yeah for sure I want to do it. I'm ready."

In my mind, this jump was going to be something we talked about for a long time and I wanted to prove to myself that I could do it on the first try.

## Luke ("Dingo")

I did not want him to go through with it! For me it was scary, and I was scared for him, but I didn't speak up enough! After the ramp was all built up, and I was actually looking at the jump, in my mind I was saying, This is fucking crazy! Especially the fact that he was going to send it over the road.

In the movies and the magazines, I saw it all the time, but those guys were professionals. We were good but we were still kids. I knew I was not at that standard to take on something like that.

I told Josh, "You don't have to do this."

But he had already made up his mind that he was going to go through with it, and I knew that he would.

I stood there for a second mentally preparing myself with the boys holding tightly onto my hands. They were going to pull me forwards and do the slingshot action to propel me faster onto the ramp. We practiced that action all afternoon, but now we were about to do it for real. There was no room for error with this jump. It was 100 percent commitment— every detail and every aspect had been well thought out. There was no plan B if anything went wrong. I felt like I didn't need a plan B because I was sure I had everything right.

I took one deep breath then leant backwards, and at the same time, the boys started pulling me forward. Next they got their speed up, and then *whooosh*, they did their slingshot action, and I was off speeding along the run-in and onto the ramp.

I thought, *Okay, the board is in the right spot.*

I heard the snow underneath my feet. It wasn't soft. Instead it was iced up and really smooth. I could hear the *ssshhhhhh* noise underneath my board and the wind in my face. I quickly glanced to my left and saw my friends watching me, and then I looked straight ahead because I had to keep my tunnel vision on the ramp and focus on what was in front of me.

In my past, if it was a new jump and it was quite a big distance, I pulled out of it right at the last moment and I would become really pissed off with myself for doing that. This time I was determined to follow through.

I said to myself, "No, I'm going to do it. I'm going to stick to it and get past my fear."

As soon as I went past the point of no return, I thought, *Yes! I've done it! I've committed!*

And you know, even at that point, I thought for a split second that I would pull out of it. But I didn't.

Then, as I came at the jump, I heard everything—especially the wind—and then I felt my feet hit the ramp and I knew straight away that everything was going to go wrong. The transition between the run-in and the ramp was too harsh and too pitched; it needed to be flatter. I hit the ramp with so much speed that my knees couldn't take the impact and they collapsed. I didn't land on my butt; I squatted and all my weight went down my legs and transferred into my heels.

Anyone who has snowboarded before knows that if they leave a jump with their heels dug into the ground, that once they leave the lip, they will turn upside down and start spinning and flipping backwards. That is exactly what happened to me. My weight transferred, my heels dug into the ground, and I flew off the lip, which made me spin upside down. I knew it was game over straight away. I was done and I had just ruined everything.

I looked at the road and felt all this noise around me—and the wind—*ssshhhhhhuuup*. And then, there was complete silence. I was upside down in the air in complete silence and I knew I had only seconds before I hit the road. Everything was happening so quickly but in that short space of time, there were a thousand thoughts spinning around in my mind.

Next I looked at the road and thought, *Don't hit the road! Don't hit the road, because whatever you look at is what you hit.*

So, with that in mind, of course I tried to do everything I could to turn myself right-side up and not hit the road. I started doing circles with my arms—the same action people do when they wind down a car window real quick. I hoped that action would bring my body around, so I tried to throw my legs underneath me. If I landed on my legs, at worst, I'd break my legs and I would rather break my legs than break my head!

Nothing I did was working. I was still upside-down and was coming at the road, and I was really freaking out and panicked at this point. I was still struggling to correct myself.

I thought, *God, what the fuck's going on? This is all wrong.*

Another part of me said, *Keep calm, keep calm, keep calm.*

I knew if I hit the road rigid I could break everything. If I hit the road soft I could distribute the weight of the impact to go right through my entire body instead of localizing it in just one spot, and I would probably break nothing at all. It was pretty obvious that wasn't going to be the case for me because I was coming in too fast and I was going to hit the road hard, and worst of all my head was coming in first.

Then I heard something.

I heard a voice say, "It's okay. You're fine, we're going to make sure that you survive this."

I just thought this was the voice in my head and I didn't recognize it at the time. The information about it came out in a hypnosis session about three months after the accident as part of my alternative rehabilitation therapy. I realized then the voice I heard was my grandfather's—my mum's dad. I was really close to him before he died. Hearing his voice and the words that he said changed everything, even when I was upside-down in the air about to slam onto the road at any given second.

I started to calm down and relax. I knew I was still going to hit the road even though I couldn't see it coming because it was behind me, but I knew I was going to be okay.

My last thoughts just before I hit the road were, *Don't hit your head, don't hit your head! Your mum is going to kill you if you hit your head.*

I made one last effort to bring my feet underneath me. At least if I landed on my hands or knees, I'd break those or break my legs so my head and back would be safe. But I was out of time.

Just before I hit the road, I heard grandfather's voice again saying, "Just stay calm, we're going to help you. We're going to make sure you are alright."

I relaxed then and calmed myself down, and said, "Alright, here it goes…"

And then I shut my eyes and just as I pulled my chin in, BANG! Straight in my neck.

I felt the violent impact of my neck as it hit the road and everything just went black. I wasn't knocked out though because I was still conscious. I was also still relaxed and calm at that point because when I knew that I couldn't do anything about it. That's when I realized that everything I control is completely gone and that I cannot control anything that was going to happen. The best thing I could do was relax and let my body go limp.

I felt my chin hit my chest at the top of my breastbone. My knees came up and hit my ears and head. Then I heard the metal edges of my board hit the asphalt road. In turn, that threw my legs the wrong way, and they went in the other direction and came up underneath me, which caused me to bounce backwards. Then I felt the back of my head hit in between my shoulder blades. I heard the plastic of my helmet hit the plastic guard that was over my back and straight away I heard the explosion of my neck snap. It all happened so fast and it was over in about two seconds, but they were the longest two seconds imaginable.

The best way to describe it is when a person tumbles backwards down a hill or a flight of stairs head first and their body rolls over the top and flings their legs up in the air, and then their legs circle down, come underneath them, and they bounce backwards off of their legs. I was glad I came to a pretty quick stop because it was a very violent impact and I couldn't believe that I wasn't knocked out, but was fully conscious and aware of everything going on around me.

As I lay there, these airy sounds came out my mouth. I tried to breathe but I couldn't breathe properly because I was having trouble figuring out which way the air had to go. At first I thought I was screaming, but it was just the air in my lungs trying to come out.

I was saying to myself, *I'm still alive, I'm alive, but I was also thinking, What am I going to do? This doesn't happen to me—this happens to someone else.*

But it did happen to me.

I just lay there saying to myself, *Fuck! I have just completely ruined my whole life. A split second ago I was healthy—now look at what I've done.*

I was still aware of everything going on around me at this point. I could hear my mates running down the road as their snow boots pounded on the road surface as well as others who ran through the snow to get to me.

The one thing I remember the most was Daniel screaming my name, "Josh... Josh!"

I never heard him scream so loud!

Daniel got to me first because he and Simon were standing on the road at the end of the jump, so I landed almost right at their feet. I was about 20-30 feet away from them.

## Daniel

I stood between the hairpin in the road and the jump. I thought this spot was the best position to take a sequence photograph because I could capture and frame the entire shot as Woody (Josh) came off the jump to being airborne for a few seconds before making it to the landing.

I watched Dingo slingshot Woody into the jump and he looked good for speed in his approach, so I held down the button and the lens began to open and close several times. As Woody left the lip I froze and things slowed down in my mind as I viewed him through the camera; he drifted back and became more and more inverted as he came closer to the road.

My heart raced as he hit the road, and I panicked and dropped the camera and sprinted to get to him. I thought he was dead by the way he bounced like ragdoll and the way that his legs bent over his head. Adrenaline raced through my veins as I shouted out, "Josh... Josh!" while I ran to him.

As I made it to him on the side of the road at the edge of the snow, people crowded around us. All I wanted was a response from him and it was good to see he was conscious.

I knelt down beside him, and Dingo was on the other side and yelled, "Back up and give him some room."

People moved back and everybody said, "Don't move him."

I asked Woody if he was okay; he looked like he wasn't in too much pain at this stage.

He looked at me and said, "Well, that wasn't worth it. I guess I won't be going to the pub now." .

I boycotted answering that statement. I said, "You'll be alright mate." But I wasn't sure if I believed what I was saying. I was just trying to reassure Woody he would be okay.

Two of the boys were beside me at this point—Daniel and Luke ("Dingo").

I said to them, "Don't touch me, don't touch me, I've broken my neck."

I could see they were both panicked. Daniel was very upset and distraught since they both just witnessed the worst possible outcome for this jump and there was a possibility that I could have still died. Daniel managed to pull himself together enough to send one of the boys straight up to the medical centre for help.

I looked at both Daniel and Dingo and I kept repeating, "Don't move me, don't move me 'cause I've broken my neck."

I knew if I was going to be as good as possible, I couldn't move a single inch. I was in so much agony that it actually felt like my spine snapped in half and was poking out through my chest. It wasn't, but it certainly felt like it. I even asked Dingo to touch my chest so I could know how bad it was.

I said to him, "Can you touch my chest? Can you see if my spine's hanging out my chest?"

Before Dingo answered me, I already thought, I've got to make sure. If it is, I'll give up right now. If its not, then I'll just hold on.

He touched my chest and said to me, "No, no, you're fine."

## Daniel

Seeing your best mate lying twisted on the road, I had to say anything to give him hope. Woody seemed to keep his wits about him, which made me less of a mess, but I was still a wreck.

He threw out one-liners such as, "Looks like we're not going to the pub tonight".

I replied, "We'll make it another time."

Then, I pulled out my phone and dialed 000 and explained to the emergency operator where we were and what happened. My voice shuddered as I spoke and I fought back tears. I didn't want to cry, especially in front of Woody, because I didn't want him to get anymore upset than he already was.

It was a quick phone call and I really can't remember what was said. I just wanted to get back to Woody.

That was the moment I started going in and out of shock a bit. I started getting cold and going stiff. My neck started going into spasms and it was wobbling about like a bobble-head doll because there wasn't anything holding it in place since it snapped on the impact. To help me, Dingo got behind me and gently placed his hands on either side of my ears and wrapped his hands around my head, which came from the back of my skull to the front of my face as he cradled my head to keep it as still as possible.

## Luke ("Dingo")

My emotions surged through my body. I thought, Holy fuck, he has just died!

I was at the top of the ramp when it happened and then I just started running down to get to him. By the time I got to where he was lying, I saw he was alive but it was obvious he was in a serious condition. I knew that there was major damage to Josh's body.

Josh said, "Don't touch me, don't touch me, I've broken my neck."

I almost wanted him to repeat the words because I couldn't believe what he had just said. This was the worst possible outcome. I knew that in this situation his neck should not move in case it caused further injury or even death, so I carefully placed my hands on the side of his head and just cradled his head in my hands and I did not let it move!

Dingo was so good at keeping my neck from wobbling and cradling my head that my body started to relax and the pain started to go away. The problem with that was my tongue became really loose and I could feel it sliding backwards down my throat. I could feel my body shutting down again and I couldn't stop it.

I thought, *Stop it, you've got to stop it. You're going through enough.*

Daniel must have realized my airways were becoming jammed and he tried to grab my tongue and pull it down. He was able to bring it forward and hold onto it. That one action from him gave me enough energy to be able to breathe normally again.

## Daniel

As I knelt down beside him, he started to shake from the pain and said to me that he couldn't feel his legs. Hearing him say that killed me but I just reassured him it would be okay and told him the ambulance was on its way. He kept slipping in and out of consciousness for a few seconds at a time and I kept talking to him to keep him awake so I had peace of mind that he was alive.

The worst moments were there on the ground, especially when he shut his eyes. I kept calling his name and he came to again and looked at me. Then, his airways got blocked and I pulled his tongue to one side to clear his mouth. It was all I could do because we knew we couldn't move him. Otherwise, I would have carried him to the medical centre myself. I had a mixture of emotions sitting beside him; I was scared and felt helpless as we waited for the ambulance to arrive.

I said to Daniel, "Ring mum, ring mum. She'll fix it. She'll make sure that I go to the right person."

He called my mum at her home. I could hear him on the phone next to me, but I couldn't move my head to look at him. I could just see him in the corner of my peripheral vision. He was walking around in circles as he was talking to her on the phone.

He kept saying, "Kay, I'm so sorry, I'm so sorry."

I could hear mum asking him questions, and then I felt the pain start to go and I drifted off again.

## Daniel

I stepped away from Josh and dialed his mum Kay's number. That's when I started crying.

I thought, How the fuck am I going to explain this to her?

Kay was very close to me. She was my second mum.

She answered the phone and I sobbed, "Josh has been in an accident."

She yelled, "Is he okay? What happened?"

I must have scared the shit out of her because I didn't know if Josh was going to make it or not and I was a mess on the phone. I can't remember what was said. Kay was prying information from my brain that was broken from witnessing what was the worst thing I'd ever seen at 18 years of age. I made it back to Woody with tears in my eyes. He was shaking from pain and I told him again that it wouldn't be long before the ambulance arrived.

## Kay

It was just after 3:40 p.m. I was on the work phone in my home office chatting to a friend in the USA when the home phone rang. Given that it was only Josh's friends who rang that number, I nearly didn't answer it, but something told me I better get it.

I picked up the phone and heard Daniel's panicked voice on the other end. He cried the words that Josh just had a terrible accident. Through his sobbing, Daniel told me that Josh was really badly injured from a jump that went wrong. He said Josh was lying on a snow road after he crashed neck first onto an asphalt road while attempting to jump it. For some reason, and I will never know why, I didn't panic. I was extremely calm, and I simply asked Daniel if Josh was conscious.

He answered, "Yes."

Then I asked him if Josh knew where he was.

Daniel sobbed, "Yes."

I said to Daniel, "Great, we have something to work with."

I have no idea why I said that.

At least I knew Josh was conscious and he knew where he was, so to be honest, I thought he wasn't that badly injured. At this stage, the Ski Patrol hadn't gotten to Josh, even though their medical centre was less than two minutes away. The next people I needed to speak to were the medical team at this resort's medical centre to find out the extent of Josh's injuries and how they were going to treat them.

And then I felt a strange sensation. I felt my soul leave my body. It came out from my mouth, like air quietly rising from inside my body, and passed through my lips—*haaaaaahhh*. I looked down at myself—I saw my body from above.

It was like my body needed a break, just for a second, to be relieved from all of the trauma and everything that was going on for a brief moment. The weirdest part of all this was that it was the most alive I had ever felt, yet I could feel the life slipping out of me. Right in that moment I realized what death really was and I realized how precious life really was. I knew my body was dying. I could feel my life slipping away and my body shutting down.

I desperately tried to stay awake, and it was the biggest, scariest, reality experience I ever went through, as I just lay there thinking, *I had everything and I just threw it all away.*

There was no pause-stop-rewind, no going back; I could do nothing to change it. This was all happening right now. Honestly, in that moment, it would have been so easy to close my eyes and give in to it—just let my life quietly slip away. I had the choice right then to either close my eyes to let go and die, or to stay awake, stay with it, and live. I chose to do that—live!

Then I came back into myself. I was back in my body.

I talked to myself and tried to stay awake because I knew that if I let myself drift off to sleep, then that would be it, and I might not wake up again.

Some of the boys tried to stabilize me as much as possible by packing snow around my back. I was on my left side; my left arm was trapped underneath my back as I lay on my shoulder. My neck dropped and my head was slightly twisted, so it looked like I dislocated my head off my shoulder.

My legs twisted around in the opposite direction to my body and my butt was on the ground, as well as my heels because the board was still attached to my feet. The boys didn't take my board off because they didn't want to move me at all. I still remember feeling the snow underneath me was so cold, but I didn't dare move in case I damaged my body even more than it already was.

So I lay there in the cold snow, completely twisted like a pretzel for 20-25 minutes until the medical centre staff arrived. Apparently, they thought it was a road accident so they had to load every single piece of life saving equipment into the ambulance before leaving the centre to come to me, which is what took them so long.

When the medical staff finally arrived, the first thing I told them was that I broke my neck, so they carefully put a neck brace on me. Instantly, I felt my neck was more secure and Dingo could finally let go after 20 minutes of hanging on to and cradling my head to keep my neck from wobbling. Then, they gently rolled me out of my twisted position and I remember hearing the *szzzchup* of bindings unzipping as they pulled the straps out. I heard it but I couldn't feel it. I knew they were my bindings because that's what mine sounded like. It sounds stupid because realistically they all sound the same, but I knew they were mine that had just come undone. I looked down to see what they were doing because I didn't feel it, and they grabbed my feet and put them on the stretcher.

It was like I was completely detached from my legs, and I felt absolutely nothing. I was terrified!

I was concerned about what was going to happen on the ride back to the medical centre. I wanted Daniel in the ambulance with me but they wouldn't allow it because there wasn't enough room. They had all the life-saving equipment around me so Daniel ran next to the ambulance.

They gently loaded me into the vehicle and they slowly took off to the medical centre only a short distance away. I remember looking out the window and seeing Daniel. He had my board and his board in his hands and the boys were all standing there. Then Daniel turned and started running alongside the ambulance.

Watching him run just broke my heart, and I thought, *What the hell have I done to my friends?*

It brought tears to my eyes as I watched Daniel run next to me and as I thought about what I put him through.

## Daniel

The ambulance arrived and they prepped Woody on a stretcher. He kept yelling out my name and I reassured him I was there because I was standing out of his view. As soon as they had him on the stretcher, he was loaded into the ambulance and they took off to the medical centre.

I ran beside the ambulance looking in at Woody just lying there, and I didn't know if he was going to make it and if this was the last time I would see him alive.

The ride from the crash site to the medical centre was only minutes away. It took about three or four minutes to get there because they had to drive slow to keep me stable, since any sudden movements could see me in more trouble than I already was. When I arrived at the medical centre and the staff unloaded me from the ambulance, the first thing I saw was the boys all lined up outside.

## Daniel

Half-way to the medical centre, I saw my dad coming towards me, and I just broke down. He heard about the accident and I explained to him what happened in the last half hour but it probably poured out like a mess of random words. He took me to the medical centre and I saw all the boys were already there. We were all stressed and very worried about Woody.

All I could think was, Is he still alive? Will he make it?

I felt guilty and questioned myself, Why didn't I do this and why didn't I do that? I should have knocked the jump down. What if we picked another location?

All this shit rattled me while we waited to hear from the medical staff about how he was doing.

As the medical staff brought me into the building, the boys were inside waiting for me, and their faces all looked as white as the snow outside. Then I drifted off for a short while because I don't remember what happened right after being brought inside. I do remember my neck was absolutely killing me. I felt like I wanted to stretch out and that I wanted to move around, even through all the pain I was in. I knew I had to stay as still as possible because I could feel my body shutting down majorly by this stage.

They took x-rays and MRIs, and they had to gavage me while I was still awake. They put tubes down my throat because they didn't think I would survive the helicopter ride, and they were definitely sure I wouldn't survive the four-hour ambulance ride to the nearest major hospital that could handle this kind of trauma. I remember feeling the tube slide down my throat, and I had to keep my neck still, which wasn't too difficult, because they left the neck brace on me to keep my neck from wobbling.

They said to me, "Okay, we need to put another tube down your nose."

This was a bit smaller than the size of a pen. It tickled my nose like crazy and I sighed out, *aaaahhh*. I just wanted to shake it.

They said, "You have to sniff this."

I told them, "You're kidding me. I've gone through enough and now I have to do this?"

It was worse than torture.

They kept trying to get it down my nose and I had to sniff at the same time to help the tube slide down, and it was so uncomfortable. I could feel something like sand in my neck. I realized it was the bones grinding on each other and I felt chunks of bone falling off. They might have been miniscule in size, but for me it felt like massive chunks, and every time I sniffed, I tensed my neck. I remember trying to get the tube down with little sniffs—*fff, fff, fff*—like that. I kept trying and sniffing, and trying and sniffing, and then it all became too much and I passed out.

My next memory was as I came out of the medical centre securely strapped up on a stretcher, and I was completely wrapped up with only my face exposed. I could see there were about 30 of my mates that I knew from the Alpine resorts standing around with my coach and a couple of my old coaches, and there were Daniel and Dingo and all the boys.

I heard Dingo say, "Geez mate, they've shut the whole mountain off for you."

The main access road to the village and all the hotels and restaurants was completely shut off. The mountain was crowded. It was the start of the school term holidays, and the start of the snow season. Being a Sunday, the resort was running at capacity. There were thousands of skiers on the mountain during the day and now with the main road access shut down, no one was able to get on or off the mountain.

## Luke ("Dingo")

I did not get to speak with Josh before he was loaded into the chopper that took him to the major trauma hospital in Melbourne. When the medics brought him out at this time it was all so crazy.

The whole mountain was shut down!

I called out to Josh, "Geez mate, they've shut the whole mountain down for you."

I don't know if he heard me or not. I stood there with the rest of the boys and we watched the medics load him in the chopper.

My thoughts were, I hope my bloody friend doesn't die on the way there!

It was after 5:30 p.m. by then, which made me a bit concerned because they start shutting the mountain down around that time and they still had to bring the helicopter in to lift me off to hospital. I looked around and I saw thousands of people behind a roped off area.

I thought, *Nah, nah I'm not that bad.*

I even commented to one of the Ski Patrollers, "I'm not that bad, get me out, I'll walk across."

He just said, "Mate, you're not going to be walking anywhere—you can't move your legs."

## Daniel

We waited a while as they assessed how damaged his body was and decided on how to best treat his injuries. We were finally told he was going to be flown to the major spinal care hospital in Melbourne, so we waited to see Woody before he got loaded into the chopper.

When he came out of the medical centre, we couldn't get in close enough to see him. He was wrapped up on a stretcher and the medical staff were moving him quickly across the snow to get him on the chopper so they could lift off because the weather had turned and visibility on the mountain became really poor.

We were left waiting there at the medical centre with our thoughts and hoping for anything other than the worst.

I remember dad saying, "Daniel, let's go home."

But I didn't want to. I said I wanted to stay with the boys because we'd all been through the same thing, and we all felt the same and understood each other. For me, it was a better environment to be with the rest of the boys. Not a lot was said that evening as we sat in our apartment at the resort, but we were all looking out for each other and we didn't want to think of the worst that could happen to Josh, though we stressed about it!

The medical guys picked me up and carried me across the road onto the snow and they gently slid me across to where the helicopter was waiting.

I could hear the sounds of the helicopter and I thought, *This is not all for me; this can't just be all for me.*

I felt completely guilty, which is why I kept persisting to the medical staff to let me get out and walk.

## Kay

When someone is seriously injured on the mountain, there are two options for getting treatment. The first is to transport the injured person down the mountain to the local hospital. The second option is by helicopter, which is how those that are seriously injured are flown into the major city centre where there are various trauma hospitals. In my mind, flying Josh back to Melbourne was the best option. There were better-equipped trauma hospitals in the city.

Josh had private health insurance, which included emergency evacuation. Initially when I rang the medical centre, they couldn't tell me anything—they were still evaluating Josh. I asked them to fly him back to Melbourne because honestly I didn't want to make the almost three-hour drive to the community hospital.

At that stage we still had no idea exactly what had happened to Josh or the extent of his injuries. My sister Wendy arrived home at that moment since she was visiting our mother at her home down the coast for the weekend.

Just before I was loaded into the helicopter, I had a real feeling of loneliness. I knew I wasn't with my friends anymore, and I only had the helicopter medics with me. That's when it started getting scary. I was on my own and I didn't have anyone I knew.

# Kay

Finally at around 5:45 p.m. they told me they were flying Josh by emergency medical evacuation to one of the specialist trauma hospitals in Melbourne. I was relieved that a decision had finally been made and they were taking action. I said to Wendy that Josh must have hurt his back in the accident because they were sending him to the hospital, which I knew was a spinal injury and major trauma hospital.

I still wasn't sure about the extent of Josh's injury. Truthfully, I was relieved he was coming back to Melbourne for treatment. I rang Josh's father Garry and arranged to meet him at the hospital.

The weather turned real nasty and visibility was so minimal that the helicopter pilot wasn't even sure if he would be able to take off safely. That's when my mate Chrisso's dad jumped on his Ski-Doo snowmobile, slowly riding it up the mountain with its bright lights on so it could act as a beacon for the helicopter to follow him by hovering close to the ground to get to the top of the run. That way, the helicopter safely cleared the path of the chairlifts and any other unforeseen obstructions.

I could hear the helicopter blades spinning faster and we were going to lift off any second. I started getting upset, but I don't remember if I cried.

The pilot turned around and said to me, "Don't worry mate, you'll be fine."

I yelled back to him, "Yeah, easy for you to say, you're not the one with a broken neck."

Then the helicopter lifted off the mountain and I was on my way to the spinal care hospital.

# Wendy

While I was driving back home after having spent the day visiting my mother when my phone rang. I looked at the screen to see who it was and Kay's number was displayed, so I answered her call and to my surprise, she immediately hung up on me.

I called her right back and said, "What's the matter? You didn't tell me what you want."

She sounded a bit distressed and said, "You need to come home."

I told her I would be there in about 10 minutes and hung up. I was surprised Kay was home because she wasn't due to fly in until the next day since she was over in Perth working.

I pulled up outside our home, jumped out of the car, and rushed straight in. I no sooner opened the front door when Kay told me Josh had a terrible accident up at the ski resort and he was being flown by helicopter to the major spinal care hospital across town.

"Spinal care hospital? Why is he being sent to the spinal care hospital?" I questioned.

Kay said the medical team up at the ski resort decided that Josh was too injured to be treated locally, so they flew him to the trauma hospital down here. There was initially some concern getting the helicopter off the mountain because the visibility became limited due to the bad weather. The greater concern, however, was if they couldn't get the helicopter off the mountain, Josh would have had to be transferred by ambulance—at least a three-hour drive and in the serious condition Josh was in, the medical team were not confident he would have survived that trip.

# Chapter 2

# Fly to Survive

## The most alive I've ever felt was when I was dying.

I was in the helicopter as it lifted off the mountain, and I was on my way to the hospital with just the medics on board with me. As much support as they gave me, I felt like I was on my own because this was the most scary and unsure time of my entire life and I was going through it alone.

I must have passed out because I don't know what happened to me in the helicopter when it was in the air. I could have been awake the whole time I was in the helicopter, but I just don't remember or have any memory of the flight once it lifted off the mountain.

The next memory I had was when we landed at the hospital.

### Kay

Wendy and I didn't even know how to get to the hospital—it was across town from where we lived. We finally managed to get through all the traffic and arrived there just as the helicopter hovered overhead preparing to land. We went straight to emergency, where to our surprise we were taken to a private waiting room. Wendy and I were relieved; emergency rooms are not our favourite places. Still neither of us realized the urgency of the situation. Josh's father Garry arrived and then a nurse asked all of us to go with them as Josh was brought into the hospital.

I knew Daniel already rang my mum. I wasn't sure if she knew the extent of my injuries or if she had enough time to drive over and be at the hospital for when I arrived. I thought that even though I was at the hospital and about to be unloaded from the helicopter and be taken inside, there might not be any of my family there to meet me and help me get through the fear and uncertainty I was experiencing.

The medics took me out of the helicopter and put me onto the landing. I was on the stretcher and strapped on very tightly and I felt the lights on my face and the warmth of the lights because they were very bright.

Then I heard voices; I heard my mum's, dad's, and Aunty Wendy's voices.

I was so relieved to know my family was right there and I thought, *Geez, they got here quick.*

I was confused at that point and didn't really understand everything that was happening to me. Then, when I saw mum and dad, I felt all this emotion come over me. It was overwhelming and then it hit me really hard—the reality of what I'd done. It was just so scary because the most confronting thing I ever faced in my life now stared me in the face. I couldn't feel my legs, I couldn't feel much of my body at all, and I didn't know if I was going to ever walk again. It was the reality of knowing I snapped my neck in half and just from that reality alone I changed my whole destiny.

I knew that one mistake when I came off the jump and was upside down in the air coming at the road head first—that one small mistake in a split second of time—completely changed everything in my life as I knew it.

When I finally saw mum, dad, Aunty Wendy, and the worried looks on each of their faces, I felt terrible for them having to see me arrive at the hospital on a stretcher all covered up. I didn't want them to be worried about me, but I knew that I was in a situation that I couldn't control. I was emotionally overwhelmed by the whole scene so I tried to diffuse the intensity of the situation by making them laugh.

I said to them, "You know I've sort of been seeing three different girls at the same time, so can you make sure they don't all come into the hospital at once? I don't want a cat fight happening in here!"

Dad said to the hospital staff, "Oh he mustn't be that bad—he's a bit of a drama queen."

## Kay

The doctors must have thought that Garry and I were mad because we both agreed there wasn't much wrong with Josh if all he was worried about was these girls that he was dating would come in to see him at the same time! We truly had no idea what had happened.

I was taken into emergency so the doctors could examine me and determine the full extent of my injuries. I was put through more rigorous examinations, poking, and prodding all around my body, x-rays, and MRIs. I didn't think it was ever going to end.

Mum, dad, Aunty Wendy, and my stepbrother Andrew came into the room just as I was being hooked up to machines that monitored my heart and body rhythms.

## Wendy

I walked into the emergency department where they placed Josh in a room. It was hard for me to see him lying there. He had every possible tube in him and around him, and he was hooked up to all sorts of monitors.

It was quite shocking and we still didn't know the extent of his injuries. The doctors were concerned that Josh didn't have feeling in his legs and certain parts of his body weren't responding to touch, so they prepared him for x-rays and MRIs to get a better idea of what they were dealing with.

I was still joking around with everyone at that stage when mum, dad, Aunty Wendy, Andrew, and my family didn't know what was going on.

Mum said, "Oh it's good we can see Josh's heartbeat."

We all didn't know it at the time but the doctors explained to us later that the only reason mum could see my heartbeat so well was because except for my heart and my brain, all my muscles were completely paralyzed, and so my body muscle biorhythms weren't registering any movement or rhythm.

## Kay

About three hours later around 9:30 p.m. the nurse came and collected Garry and I and took us into the emergency room. There were several doctors still working on Josh, who was still conscious and cracking jokes. One of the doctors walked over next to us and said they managed to stabilize Josh and were going to do more x-rays and MRIs on him, They needed to know the situation because at that stage they established that Josh couldn't feel anything below the C5 vertebrae and they needed a clearer picture of what damage sustained that area.

The doctor said that he would let us know what showed up in the scans as soon as they were done and that we could expect the process to take a bit of time so we should find a comfortable place to wait. We walked out and went back to the private waiting room and thought the doctors were being thorough with their examination.

I just sat down when the messages to my head started. The messages were really clear and urgent: "Massage Josh's fingers, hands, toes, and feet. There are people around you that will help you and never give up!"

I told Wendy I was hearing messages to start massaging Josh's body.

I said to her, "I must be going crazy. Where are these messages coming from?"

The messages were unrelenting and came over and over again. At that point I had no idea what they meant.

I was still in the emergency department with a group of doctors examining me. Tubes, tubes, and more tubes were all over me and connected to several monitors. I had a feeding tube fitted and it brought back old memories for mum. She said it was like seeing me when I was a baby because there were some complications with my birth and I was placed in the Special Care unit for the first two weeks of my life, and at that point I also had a feeding tube to get the nutrients into me.

Now 18 years later, it was the same deal. The doctors wanted to take me for more x-rays and MRIs. They were going through a process of elimination so that they knew exactly what they were dealing with and at this stage I was mentally so over it already. I just wanted to know myself what damage I had done and what they were going to do about it.

The process took so long that I drifted off to sleep. I was totally exhausted by this stage and I just wanted to be taken upstairs and be put in a bed in a ward so I could sleep. Finally, the doctors finished with all the scans and they took me to ICU and placed me in a bed. They said my family was still waiting there but they could come in to say goodnight to me and then they could go home.

# Kay

It was about 2:00 a.m. when Garry and I were called to meet with the doctors. Finally, we would learn what was going on with Josh. Wendy came in with us. My immediate thought was that they were going to tell us they were keeping him overnight and then we could take him home.

We were taken to a private consulting room where we were introduced to a specialist doctor. He calmly told us that Josh was badly injured and he had broken his neck, which severely crushed his spinal cord. He mentioned C5, C6, C7, and T1 complete; he even repeated it to make sure it sunk in Josh was a high-level quadriplegic.

Josh was complete. What did that mean?

The doctor's language was confusing and we were so exhausted but still tried to make sense of it all. The doctor explained that meant Josh was paralyzed from the injury from the point in his neck downwards.

Again he repeated, "He has badly crushed his spinal cord, so he'll never walk again. There is a chance he may have limited use of one of his arms. It is to early to say, but it is likely he will never get out of bed."

I thought, How can this doctor make assumptions about Josh's future so quickly?

He said Josh might have a small arm movement but we should not expect too much. I told him that Josh was an elite athlete, and therefore his mind was tough. He worked through serious injuries before this, so he had fantastic tolerance for pain and given time he would walk.

The doctor replied, "Ms. Wood, the sooner you accept your son's condition, the better off he will be. Accept that he will never walk again and that he may not even get out of bed."

I retorted, "My son is tough. He will walk, and he will never accept that he can't walk again and I won't accept it either! You don't know Josh and you don't know me! My son will walk again!"

The doctor turned to me and coolly said, "That's the problem— mothers like you. The sooner you accept that your son will never walk again, the better off you'll both be."

At that moment I could have ripped out that doctor's heart.

As I fought to remain calm, I said to him, "My son will never accept your diagnosis and neither will I."

With that he said, "I feel sorry for your son. If you don't accept my prognosis, he will have a sad life."

He went on to inform us that surgery would be scheduled sometime in those next few days to perform the fusion of Josh's broken vertebrae. They planned to take a piece of bone from his hip and fuse the C6 and C7 vertebrae, and remove the shattered vertebrae from his cord.

We asked him and Josh's other doctors not to tell Josh that his spinal cord was crushed and only that his neck was broken until after the operation, and not to tell him unless either Garry or I were present. At this stage there was still a chance that Josh could die, so we wanted everyone to be calm and remain confident that he would be okay.

The doctor said we could see Josh in ICU. Although I was numb with shock, my mind was racing as the adrenaline pumped through my body. I just wanted to wake up and find out that this was all a dream. I felt sick at the thought of Josh's injuries because this wasn't meant to happen to my boy. He was special, protected, and so vibrant—how could he cope with such an injury?

Through all this time, the one thing I was totally positive about was that Josh was going to get better and he was going to walk again! I was so frightened, but I knew if Josh saw us upset or even worried, he would get scared and then only God knew what would happen. No matter how hard it was, we had to remain positive and upbeat.

Garry, Wendy, and I arrived at ICU around 3:00 a.m. We were all emotionally exhausted by this time. Josh was all wired up to the various machines and he looked exhausted. They gave him sedatives to settle him down for the night and he was already drifting off to sleep. We planned to wait until after the operation to tell Josh about the extent of his injuries because the medical team didn't know if he was going to live.

We just said to him, "You really have to stay strong. You're having an operation probably on Monday or Tuesday and it will be huge. The doctors are going to rebuild your vertebrae."

By this stage, Josh's heavy sedatives kicked in and he was too relaxed to really understand what was happening. Josh had 24-hour one-on-one care, and even though the ward itself was very old, the nursing staff was very attentive and thorough with him. I felt confident that he was safe there, but we didn't stay long because Josh was exhausted and was drifting in and out of sleep. We knew he was stable, and we felt it was best to leave him to rest so we left to go home. We were all so mentally drained and were still operating in disbelief of what we just went through during those past hours. I don't know how many times we just wanted to wake up from that nightmare.

## Wendy

It was after 3 a.m. by now and Kay, Garry, and myself said goodnight to Josh in ICU. I couldn't believe what we were experiencing. My sister was just told that her only child was a complete quadriplegic and he would never walk again. It was just shocking news. I couldn't believe it myself.

I even said to one of the nurses, "It's a bit like a dream, really. I hope somebody wakes me up."

The nurse turned around and quite abruptly said to me, "It's not a dream—it's real life. You have to deal with it."

With a remark like that, I wondered just what we were in for. I looked at Josh and I was satisfied that he would get some sleep because the nurses sedated him well and he was already nodding off as we said goodbye.

I went to the hospital with Kay in her car—a navy-blue MX5. I didn't think Kay was in any position to drive, so I said I would drive us home. Kay wouldn't have it. She said she needed something to do to get her mind off the experience of the past several hours, so I gave in and let her drive.

Kay loved having this car. Just after Josh left home, she bought it as a present for herself and she always drove with the roof down. There was no exception that night, so there we both were in the middle of winter, freezing as it was at 3:30 a.m. in a car with the roof down and the heater at full throttle. I calmly gave her simple directions—turn left here, stop here, go right—for the 30-minute drive home.

The ICU building was pretty old and dated. At some stage it was added on to the hospital's main building to house the critical spinal care wards. This section of the hospital's wings and buildings were not designed very well; it was a collection of really old, outdated buildings scattered around the perimeter of the grounds that made me feel like I was in a third-world country at times. Inside in the acute spinal wards was just as bad. There were holes in the plaster and the paint was peeling off the walls in some areas. The curtains around the beds were also broken, and it felt cold and damp all the time. It was just a real downer of a place.

Really early the next morning, Andrew "Lammo" Lamerton came in to see me in ICU. Mum rang him to let him know it was okay to come in and visit me; I was only allowed to have two visitors at a time, so my family and friends waited in the waiting rooms and mum organized which two would come in next to take it in turns.

Mum arranged for all my snowboard gear to be brought into my ICU ward. Having my gear around me kept me connected to my life—connected to how I had lived and to how I would live. Just smelling my motor cross helmet—the smell of the dirt, fuel, and oil—stimulated my mind and my senses. It began to motivate me to recover so I could get back to all these sports that I lived to do. The hospital atmosphere was so dormant and uninspiring to me that the sight and smell of my gear became essential to me separating from where and how I currently was to where and how I was going to be.

## Kay

I left early in the morning for the hospital the next day. I hadn't slept at all and I just wanted to get back to see how Josh was doing. On my way over I was in contact with Daniel and his dad Geoff;

they came down from the mountain to see Josh and they brought his car back with his belongings. I arranged for them to bring Josh's snowboard to the hospital. Once it was there I took it into the ICU and placed it where he could see it.

The hospital staff said, "You can't take a snowboard into ICU."

I said, "I will do whatever it takes to give Josh the confidence that he will get his life back. The snowboard stays!"

He needed to see that his life wasn't over. I would not allow it to be removed! Not only did the snowboard make it to ICU, but also his snowboard boots, all his ripped clothing, and his motorbike gear mysteriously made it to the ICU as well—much to the aggravation of the medical team.

My other mate Paul "Dutchy" De Bruyn also came in later that day around dinnertime with his dad Bill. Mum brought him into my area and left him with me so we could chat privately while Mum left to speak with Bill. Dutchy was a six-foot four-inch Aussie Rules footballer; he was a big boy with a really athletic build. Dutchy and I were like brothers because we spent nearly every day together and we just finished VCE, our final year of high school.

We were together only the week before snowboarding and I hadn't seen him since the accident. He came in and he just looked dead inside when he saw me. I think the reality of seeing how much I changed in just one day after the accident really affected him.

I had already lost a couple of kilograms of weight in the very first day just because everything was paralyzed, which makes people look totally emaciated, almost skeletal, and extremely vulnerable. In just over two weeks I lost 26 kilograms. Mum used to say how scary it was just seeing the weight fall away. I looked very dark around my eyes and my face really sunk. Anyone who didn't know me would have thought I was a heroin addict.

My mates tried to lie because they didn't want to show their emotion, but I could see in their eyes how much it affected them; Dutchy especially, because it just tore him apart, and I hated seeing the sadness in his eyes—it really upset me.

## Kay

I didn't see Paul come out and there was only one door in and out of ICU. I knew he had to be in there somewhere so I went looking for him. I finally found him in an empty ICU room sobbing his heart out. I gave him a hug and said we just had to believe that Josh would be okay. I told him about the messages and how we had to massage Josh's feet and hands.

Every time Paul came to visit Josh after that night, he massaged Josh's hands and feet even though Josh told him to stop. Josh said it felt weird and he was uncomfortable but Paul kept on doing it. He never gave up on Josh.

Visitors were starting to stream into my room at the hospital in numbers. In the first 24 hours I had around 60 people come in to see me.

## Kay

Before I let anyone see Josh, I explained that they had to remain very positive and that they weren't to discuss Josh's cord damage or the extent of his injuries. At that stage Josh was convinced that as soon as his neck was stabilized and the vertebrae were re-constructed, he would be out of hospital. I asked everyone to massage his hands and feet. No one was going to just go in to see him and stand around doing nothing. My priority and focus was for Josh to get his life back and I knew we had to start immediately. Everyone visiting Josh had to be part of this process! If they weren't going to be part of the process, then they wouldn't be allowed to see him. Tough, but simple.

I was convinced that if Josh knew the extent of the damage, he would not survive the operation and he would just give up if he thought he had no future, or hope of ever getting out of bed, or ever walking again. I had to keep him positive and believing he was going to be all right. That was the most important role I had!

I knew that my hands were completely useless and I couldn't use my right hand enough to do anything. I'm left-handed but I couldn't use it to do everyday things like write with a pen. I couldn't even use it to eat my food, let alone scratch my nose, and it drove me mad! From day one, I did a lot of work on my hands to keep the circulation going and keep them moving. Mum massaged my hands and feet using essential oils and stuff like that. She was convinced the massaging would help send messages to my brain to keep my body stimulated and keep the muscles moving so they didn't waste away. My friends came in and massaged my feet. I was massaged for hours every day on my hands, my fingers, my arms, my feet, and my toes. I know they were just trying to help me but I hated all the touching.

One time when Dutchy was massaging my feet, I said to him, "Can you piss off? I'm sick of you touching my feet. It's uncomfortable and I don't want my mate touching my feet. It's weird."

He said to me, "Until you can kick me out of the way, I'm going to keep on massaging your feet, so get over it."

And I couldn't fight with that.

My mates came in diligently and mum said to them, "You know you have to massage his feet. You don't just go in there and stand around and do nothing, you have to do something!"

It helped because it made me want to have my own independence away from it all. The doctors and nurses told us we were wasting our time but mum didn't give a shit. She made everybody give me a massage when they came in to see me.

In the first few days when I was in ICU, my Grandma—my mum's mother—came to visit me. She's just a little short lady and she couldn't get close enough to me to give me a kiss because the bed I was in had high bars up the sides, but she kept trying to get to me and I couldn't touch her.

I only managed to pat her on the top of her head and I told her, "It's okay Dottie, everything's going to be okay, it's going to be okay, and I'm sorry I've done this to you."

It was so hard because I couldn't even hug my own family and I went through all these emotions as I thought, *How the hell am I going to fix this?*

I had all my family and friends around me, but I felt so alone and it was scary. My friends and a couple of my cousins came in once and they started crying when they saw me. I told them they're not the one with the broken neck, so they needed to get out if they were going to cry. I had to be that hard person because if I cried, I wouldn't stop, and I might not have ever had the drive to continue to look forward and never look backward.

I never saw mum cry once. Whether she did or not, I don't know. It wasn't only because she didn't want me to see her cry since she knew it would upset me; it was also because she gave me so much confidence and I saw so much belief and trust in her that I knew I was going to be okay and I was going to get back what I had lost. She didn't really have time to cry because she was concentrating on me and making sure I had the drive to keep going and never give up.

I believed that no matter how much damage there was, I was going to walk again. When I thought about my upcoming operation in the next few days, I was positive I was going to get everything back that I had lost and this was what I was thinking as I went into that operation.

## Kay

Josh really had no idea about the extent of his injury. He knew he broke his neck but he thought that once they operated, he would be back on the mountain snowboarding the next week. Everyone knew but Josh. Everyone was sworn to secrecy.

I spent those pre-operation days threatening the doctors who were insistent on telling Josh that his cord was crushed and whose opinions were that there was no hope he would ever walk again or even be able to get out of bed. He was a C5, C6, C7, and T1 complete quadriplegic and we all had to just accept it. I threatened them with everything if they told him. I knew he would never survive the operation if he knew the full extent of his injuries and that the doctors thought there was no hope for him for anything in his life but to be bedridden and dependent on everyone else to help him do the everyday things in life like dress himself, feed himself, wash and shower, and go to the toilet.

The doctors didn't recognize that Josh was an athlete and that he had worked through other injuries including an L5 fracture. They didn't want to hear that he had been under the expert care of a brilliant chiropractor for two years, which had essentially fixed the L5 injury. All they cared about was that we accepted their prognosis for Josh's benefit. That's what they believed and they were determined to have us believe the same, but I had none of it and neither did Josh.

I was happy to finally have the operation on Wednesday. My family and friends stayed later that night and they kept me feeling positive about the surgery. I thought that as soon as they operated on and stabilized my neck and fixed up the broken vertebrae, I would have some recovery time and maybe some rehab, but then I would be fine. I thought I would be snowboarding again in no time.

I was told that I was going to have major surgery to rebuild my neck, which made me feel like I had a good chance of recovery. Otherwise, what would be the point to go through all that surgery if I wasn't going to walk away?

The doctors told me it was going to be a big operation and it would take several hours to get through and repair all the damage. It sounded complicated because they planned to take bone from my right hip and use it to repair the broken vertebrae. They chiseled the bone using a hammer. It sounds crazy but that's how they did it. They needed to cut me around my neck and throat area to operate on the broken vertebrae and remove the shattered bone. They went in from just below my jaw through to the other side of my esophagus and moved everything to the side out of the way, and then, with the bone they took from my hip, they rebuilt my C6 and C7 vertebrae.

## Kay

The operation was coming up and I kept asking the doctors questions about Josh's injury. I wanted to be confident and know what to expect before he went in for surgery.

Three days after Josh's accident, I probed his Consultant Specialist with questions, when in frustration he said to me, "Look, Kay, we just don't know!"

I hugged him and told him joyfully that this was the best news we had received in three days.

I said, "Why didn't you say that to me on Sunday night?"

He couldn't answer.

## Josh's first MRI's

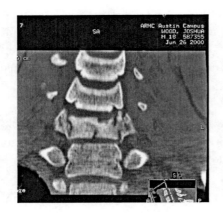 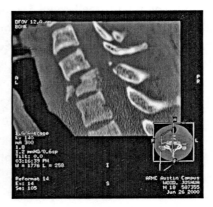

## Plate that was put in place to stabalize Josh's vertabrae

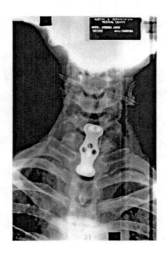

# When No Hope is Given

## Sometimes you just need to take off your shoes and walk in some grass.

### Kay
*Reflections of the night of 25 June 2000*

When I finally reached our home on the night of the accident, I was numb with shock and overwhelmed with grief. I went to my room and sat on my bed. I felt totally hopeless as to how I could possibly help Josh. But I knew if there was a way, I would find it!

I was stressed out of mind so I yelled out to God. It truly wasn't a prayer—it was more like a command: "If there is a God, I need the names of those that will help me and I need them now!"

Wow! Four names instantly exploded in my head: Simon, Paula, Dana, and John (USA). These four people didn't know it at the time, but they were the catalyst of Josh's recovery team.

### Kay

Josh was operated on Wednesday, 28 June 2000 in the late evening, which was three days after his accident. We all left the hospital to try and get some much-needed sleep because we were told the surgery would take several hours. The doctor agreed to call us once Josh was back in recovery.

The operation would remove the splintered vertebrae from in and around the spinal cord and remove some of the pressure on the cord in order to rebuild the shattered C6 and C7 vertebrae by screwing them together with the titanium plate. Bone was going to be taken from Josh's right hip to be used to rebuild the shattered vertebrae.

Firstly, the muscles would be peeled back to expose the hipbone. Some of the hipbone would then be chipped away and crushed, and then placed back over the shattered vertebrae to help it rebuild. The surgery would be performed through the side of Josh's neck and throat.

Since we had top private health insurance, I was confident we had the best team to perform this delicate surgery. The surgery was delayed by a day as we waited for some specialized software to come from the USA.

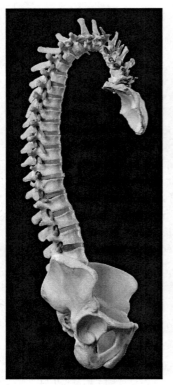

I woke up at around 3 a.m. and I couldn't move at all. I knew I had the surgery because I could feel a tingling sensation on the area around my neck where they cut into me and moved things around. There was some pain on the skin in the area they operated on, but it wasn't too bad because my body was paralyzed. At that time, I still didn't know to what degree I was paralyzed. I couldn't move any part of my body and it felt like it was being held down by restraints.

I thought, *What the hell have I done? I've obviously lost it in here and they've had to restrain me.*

All I had were these visions of me losing it in surgery and trying to belt everyone so they had to put restraints on me.

I started yelling out and the nurse came in and said, "What's wrong?"

And I said, "I need to get out of here. I need to speak to a surgeon."

She said, "Okay," and she went to get him.

I think the surgeon came in about 20 minutes later and he said to me, "What's your problem?"

He came from the left side, down at my feet and stood there.

I said, "I need to get these restraints off."

At that same time, I had all these weird thoughts flashing through my mind.

I thought, *My wallet is up there (in the apartment at the ski resort). The boys have probably found my wallet and thought it is payback time. They are probably going to rip my money out and go to the pub. I've left shit everywhere. I've got dirty clothes lying around and all my stuff is scattered through the apartment. I've got to get back up the hill; the doctors have fixed me so I'm sweet, I'm out! Okay, sorry, I have learnt my lesson—you can let me out now!*

Then the doctor said, "I've seen your history. You say you're an extreme sports person. Well, you've done the ultimate goal. You'll never walk again!"

I stayed silent for a second as I tried to process what he just said to me. I was an 18-year-old kid in a hospital. I couldn't move; I was in pain and I was frightened because I didn't even know where I was. I didn't know if I was in Melbourne or somewhere else, and I had no one with me—no family, no friends, no one.

All I knew was it was 3:30 a.m. I was alone and scared and this surgeon told me that I would never ever walk.

I said to him, "Well, you did the surgery didn't you?"

And he said, "Yes we rebuilt your neck as good as possible, but you've destroyed your neck and you'll never walk. Your legs are completely useless."

That was the most brutal thing that anyone ever said to me. If I thought I had already lost it before in the recovery room, I was wrong. Now I was going to lose it! I demanded they call my mum and get her to come in right now! They left me alone while they called mum. Those words were like an explosion that went off in my head.

The thoughts of, *What's the point of living like this if I am going to be a vegetable? And, Obviously this doctor knows because he sees it all the time. Fuck it! I need to die!*

I knew I couldn't kill myself because I couldn't move, so I thought, *I'll bring mum in. I'll just pressure her into killing me. I'll make her feel bad enough to kill me because at the end of the day it will be better for her. Then she won't have to deal with me being like this.*

Then, I had another thought, *If I can get some recovery in my hands in the next week or two, then I can use my own hands to kill myself. I can find some way to get it done if I can just get some movement back in my hands.*

I was way beyond the reach of any rational thinking at this point.

I kept saying to myself over and over again, *How the fuck am I going to kill myself? I can't even lift my damn hand to scratch my nose!*

I was on a roll, so I came up with another plan. I thought this one would definitely work. I planned to find a friend that would kill me! I remembered my stepbrother Andrew and I made a pact together. If he had a motorcycle accident (because he rode Harleys) that left him brain damaged or in a vegetative state that he couldn't move, I would help him die. And he promised to do the same for me. So I had my solution— Andrew would remember our pact and he'd help me die!

I relaxed then and thought, *Sweet, I can rely on Andrew to help me!*

I would just wait for him to come in and then I'd put the hard word on him.

## Kay

It was 3:00 a.m. when my phone rang—it was the ICU nurse.

She just said, "You need to get here quickly."

I asked if Josh was okay.

She said, "No, he's extremely distressed."

"What has happened?" I asked her.

Immediately, I realized they told Josh the news that we kept from him for those three agonizing days.

I totally lost it with her. I was very clear from the moment we knew what happened to Josh that when the time came to tell him the devastating news, both his father and I had to be present! Telling Josh while he was on his own was my worst nightmare. I felt like I had totally let Josh down! I was in total shock—I could not believe they told him while he was on his own!

By car, at that time of the morning, I was about 30 minutes from the hospital. I jumped out of bed and since it was the middle of winter, I pulled track pants over my pajamas, threw on a hoody, and raced to the hospital.

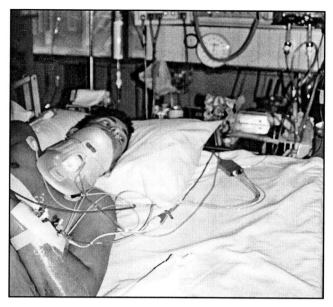

While I was waiting for mum to arrive, my thoughts had just consumed me. I wanted to die! There was no point in staying alive. What's the point in living if you can't ever move again?

*I want to die. I want to die,* This thought just kept repeating itself over and over in my mind, *I want to die. I can't live like this.*

I also kept having visions of myself being dragged into a paddock, getting shot, and then being put in a hole. That's what I felt I deserved. That's what I felt was the best option. I didn't want to be this person who they said I was going to be the rest of my life!

Then I saw mum.

She came straight to me and said, "They've told you haven't they?"

I said, "What do you mean?"

And she said, "They've told you about your injury."

I said, "Yep."

And she said, "Those bastards were never meant to say anything. They were not meant to tell you unless Dad and I were with you."

They wanted to be with me to protect me from having the reaction I had. Mum was devastated.

I said, "Mum, what's the fucking point of being like this? I'm never going to be able to do anything I want again. I've ruined my life. I've ruined my mates' lives already—seeing Dutchy so broken! I don't want to see any other mates broken like that again. Seeing one was enough!

It's too much, mum, there's no point. What's the point in living if I can't ever move again? I want to die. I want to die!"

I was always that kid who looked out the window and thought that there's a whole world to explore. I wanted to go do so many things! I was only eighteen with my whole life ahead of me and I was just told that the life I knew was gone. All gone. I was never going to walk again and all this stuff was going on in my head.

Then I said the words to mum I'm sure she'll never forget.

I said, "Mum, I can't live like this. I want you to somehow get a gun and get me into a paddock and I will kill myself."

## Kay

It was about 4:00 a.m. when I pulled up in the hospital car park. I parked the car in the closest parking spot I could find to the Spinal Care Unit. I finally reached Josh and he looked destroyed! He asked me to come close to him. I was terrified yet trying to be positive.

I said, "So you know what has happened?"

He said, "Yes!"

Before I could say anything else, Josh said to me that he wanted me to get a gun for him so he could kill himself. I cannot explain the fear that enveloped me at that moment. I have never been so scared in my life! I knew it was critical for Josh that I remain calm and not lose it, which in truth is how I felt—I had to hold it together for Josh no matter what!

As calmly as possible, I said, "You know mate, you should have died on the road Sunday, but you didn't. Something stopped you! Something in you wanted to live! I am sorry darling, but I can't let you kill yourself. I won't help you nor will anybody else. I really believe you want to live!"

He didn't answer. He was just silent. He just looked at me and it was just devastating!

I quietly said, "Josh, I know I haven't been the best mother. I always try, but I do get it wrong sometimes. But I will ask you this: Have I ever lied to you or made you a promise I haven't kept?"

He said, "No."

"So Josh, I'm not about to change now. I really believe you will walk again—I just know it! You have to believe that anything is possible!

These doctors don't know you. We've worked through some tough injuries before! Seriously Josh, I don't know what we'll do, but I will find a way. You will walk!"

At that moment I don't know whether Josh just thought, I'll go along with her, but he seemed to become calmer and less frightened!

We talked quietly together for hours. By the time we finished, Josh had set a series of goals and I made promises that we have both kept still to this day.

Mum looked me straight in the eye and said to me, "Josh, you were meant to die three days ago and you survived. You're still here. You have the strongest mind and will power, and you can still talk. There's obviously something in you that's made you survive, and if anyone's going to get anything back, it's going to be you!"

We talked for hours after that. We weren't talking about walking or anything like that, just survival, and, "You're going to come out of this as good as you can be" kind of talk.

And I thought, *Well, I can't kill myself, and mum won't kill me, and if my mates kill me, she'll end up killing them—so they definitely won't help me die.*

I looked at mum and said, "Well, I guess I've got no other option except to live, have I?"

I believed mum. I believed her because I didn't die. Maybe there was something in me that decided to not give up and live after all! To continue to talk about killing myself was just going to be a cop out and I would devastate so many people if I did. I was never going to say anything like that again! I would do whatever it took to walk again and get back what I'd lost and mum was going to help me. She would make sure I got the best treatment possible. After all that talking with mum, I was exhausted. I was in a bit of pain and I just wanted to go back to sleep and block it all out of my mind.

# Kay

After our conversation, I was mentally distraught from hearing Josh talking about wanting to kill himself or have me help him kill himself. I was never more frightened in my life or more frightened for my son! I knew the doctors would fix Josh, but they wouldn't heal him. For Josh to be mended or healed, I knew I had to build our own team of healers consisting of alternative therapists and practitioners to heal Josh. And that was exactly what I was going to do.

I knew I had to look further than what was being offered by the doctors, which was acceptance for Josh's prognosis. In their eyes, their work was done. I was sure Josh was going to be okay. He was exhausted and he wanted to sleep. I stayed with him until he dozed off and then I returned home to find and organize our alternative recovery team.

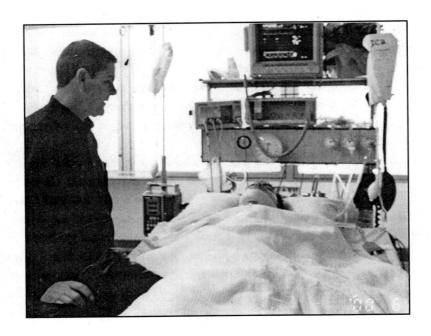

I woke up sometime later and was still in the recovery room. In the time from being so brutally told by the surgeon that I'd never walk again and talking everything over with mum—falling back asleep for a while and then waking up—there was a definite shift in my thoughts and feelings. I just wanted to get on with getting myself better.

## Kay

The night of the accident, I pleaded with Josh's doctors to allow Simon to be involved with Josh's treatment. I argued that Simon treated Josh for so many years. They trusted each other. He knew Josh inside and out and most importantly, I had total faith in Simon. The doctors said it was not possible, and that chiropractors were not allowed to practice at the hospital.

I realized it was pointless arguing with them, so I decided on a strategy that I would use for the entire time Josh would be in hospital and in rehab: I would lie!

So Simon would be Josh's Specialized Snowboard Coach!

Mum was going to speak to my chiropractor Simon. He treated me for the past two years for an L5 fracture I sustained while I snowboarded in Switzerland. I landed awkwardly on a large rock as I came off a jump. At the time, I had no feeling in my legs so I crawled through the snow to the nearest treatment facility. The impacted area on my lower back eventually settled down and I got all feeling back in my legs almost straight away. But later, the injured area kept on troubling me through chronic lower back pain.

When I came back to Australia, Simon and I developed a complete treatment plan together, including a gym program to relieve my back pain. I visited Simon twice a week over a two-year period. He consistently kept working on me and eventually sorted my back out. In fact, the irony of it all was that I walked out of Simon's surgery on 23 June 2000, just two days before my accident on the mountain.

Simon's words to me were, "Josh you have the back of an 18-year-old—well done. Two years of hard work have paid off. Go for it and have some fun."

# Kay

It was the Monday morning after Josh's accident at around 6:00 a.m.

I was still in total shock. I wasn't able to sleep and I felt like I had to do something. So I decided to go and see Simon and I hoped that he could explain to me what was going on!

I raced down to Simon's chiropractic surgery. It was located about five minutes from our home. I walked into the practice and my emotions were at breaking point.

Simon was walking down the stairs as I blurted out, "Josh has had this terrible accident."

I rambled through what happened. The poor man didn't know what to say to me. He was also in shock.

It was only the Friday before that Josh bounded out of the surgery hearing Simon say, "Your back is back to where it should be. Go have fun."

I said, "What does it mean, Simon? They say his spinal cord is crushed."

He said that before he could comment he needed to see Josh's MRIs. It was imperative that I get access to them because he needed to know what he was dealing with. We talked for a while and naturally he agreed to help us. He was so positive that Josh was strong enough and his mind was tough enough to achieve anything. Simon reiterated that although there was no question that he was tough, this would be Josh's greatest battle, but Simon was positive that Josh was up to it.

This gave me hope that anything was possible and that my son just might get his life back.

As I left the practice, Simon called me to remind me, "Kay, we need to see the MRIs."

My mission, along with everything else I had to do, was to get copies of Josh's x-rays and MRI scans. I thought it would be as easy as just asking the hospital for a copy. I was shocked to be told that I could not access any of Josh's medical records and information, because Josh was over 18 years of age and legally an adult. Therefore, only he could access them. I wasn't prepared for this. I naturally assumed that since I was his legal next of kin, I could access any information on Josh.

I contacted my financial planner at 9:00 a.m. and told him what had happened. I needed a Medical Power of Attorney document written up that day. Josh couldn't sign and I wondered how we would do it. What a nightmare! I also advised him to sell everything I owned. I was self-employed at that time, so we needed money to live on because it would be a while until I would be able to work again.

Somehow, that day the Medical Power of Attorney was produced and signed off legally. Even then, it took several days of hassling with the hospital to finally gain access to those precious MRIs and x-rays. The catch was that I had to actually copy them myself. Yet again, I was met with a complete lack of assistance from the hospital. I copied three complete sets to make sure I had enough.

Now that I finally had copied sets of Josh's MRIs, I took them to show Simon at his practice. He went through them with me. He said there was good news and bad news; whilst the cord was badly crushed, it was not severed. There seemed to be a small amount of functioning spinal cord, so the challenge was to keep it stimulated. I was so relieved that we massaged Josh's feet, toes, hands, and fingers from day one. Simon felt this needed to be done for as many hours as possible each day.

We simply worked on the premise that, "If you don't use it, you lose it". Very basic, but it became our mantra.

When Simon came into see Josh later that first week, it was his role to keep the energy flowing through Josh's badly beaten body. I wanted to use the copies I had of Josh's MRIs to get a second opinion preferably not from an Australian doctor. I knew there were specialists in America. Due to America's larger population than ours, I thought there could possibly be more specialists in the USA that had greater experience in this field. If they saw Josh's MRIs, they could pick up something new or find something the doctors here in Australia had missed. If that was the case, then it would throw some different light on the prognosis.

So my next mission was to get Josh's scans over to the USA and have a specialist look at them and give their opinion. I discussed this with Josh's medical team. They were really angry that I wanted to seek a second opinion, and even more angry that I wanted the second opinion to come from an American specialist.

They argued with me and said, "We have the same information they have, and we have the same expertise."

I counter argued that with our small population, our doctors didn't have the experience since Australia has significantly less spinal cord injuries. To have a specialist in America take a look at Josh's MRIs, I had to get the copies over there, and I knew just the two people who I could rely on to help me.

I met Dana and John, an American couple, through the Anthony Robbins Life Mastery course I did in 1999. We met at Honolulu airport while waiting in the line to board the plane to Kona. At the time, we chatted briefly and I ran into them several times over the next 10 days that I was involved in the course. We developed a friendship based on our shared experiences with Life Mastery.

I kept in touch with Dana and John since my return to Australia. I knew I could count on them both! I rang them the night of Josh's accident and Dana offered to jump on the first plane that night and fly over to Melbourne but I explained that she could better help me if she stayed in the USA and get Josh's MRIs to a specialist there so we could have a second opinion. Dana said all I had to do was send her the MRIs and she would take care of the rest.

Immediately after my prayer was answered that first night (with the names of people who could possibly help Josh recover) I phoned Dana in the USA. Speaking to her calmed me down a little. I felt that I had a new recovery team member—someone I could trust to help us.

Dana researched and located the top spinal injury specialist based at a trauma hospital in Los Angeles. I was able to send Dana a complete copied set of Josh's MRIs and x-rays for this specialist to have a look at. When she eventually met with the orthopedic surgeon at the hospital and he looked through all the copies Dana brought, he agreed with the Australian doctors' prognosis. Although this was devastating news, we just took it in our stride. We quickly realized our initial thoughts of seeking out alternative recovery therapy would be our only option for Josh's long-term recovery.

The nights were by far the worst time for me. I had all my family around me but I felt so alone.

All sorts of crazy thoughts went through my mind: *What if there is a fire in the hospital—how will I get out? Will the nurses be able to get me out or will they just leave me here to burn to death? What if someone comes in and robs me? What if someone comes in and tries to kill me?*

I lay there with my legs dead straight and I didn't know if it was my own thinking out of sheer panic and fear for my situation, or whether all the medication I was on was scrambling my brain. I couldn't feel my legs properly and I was getting messages that my legs were broken in half or they were twisted behind the back of my head, but they were dead straight. It was so scary and crazy.

My body felt like it was on fire 24/7, as though it was severely burned and the painful tingling sensation felt like someone was scratching their nails on top of my skin all the way down my body and I couldn't do anything about it. It was like torture.

I could feel the top part of my body was on fire the most because that's the area I still had the most feeling and sensation in. Still, I couldn't relieve the pain—I could never twist around and get comfortable. I had to wait every two hours for what they call *the turners* to come in and what they would do every two hours was turn me over and place me on my side—left or right—they would swap sides around or put me on my back again because I couldn't physically move myself an inch.

My chiropractor Simon was given the title of *Specialized Snowboard Coach*. Paula the psychic healer was mum's *sister-in-law* and Isabel, the spiritual healer and massage therapist, was my *cousin*. I had to give it to mum for her creative thinking! She gathered the alternative practitioners to heal me and she gave them the pseudo names and titles so they wouldn't arouse suspicion. Simon also introduced us to Jackie who was a reflexologist that worked at Simon's chiropractic practice.

They each played a very important role in my recovery program and when they combined their knowledge and their techniques together, they were very successful with getting my body to respond. I felt it was the right approach to help soothe the burning sensations my body was experiencing and to calm my mind to unscramble the scrambled messages.

Another thing about all the weird brain activity I was experiencing was my dream state. I had so many dreams and nightmares practically every time I closed my eyes. One particular dream that kept recurring was that I stood and then I'd take a few steps and I'd walk. I could so clearly see myself standing and walking perfectly fine. I kept having a recurring nightmare that I would either fall off cliffs in a car accident or slam into a tree at high speeds. When I woke up from this dream, I opened my eyes to see that I would be sitting up straight in bed! And as soon as I realized I was awake and sitting up straight, I'd fall back flat into the bed.

After this happened, it got me thinking that if I was physically sitting up straight in bed, then there were messages going to my brain

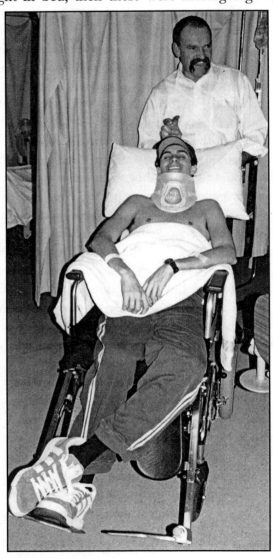

somehow—whether they were involuntary or not—there were messages creating movement. All I could think of was that I had to get off whatever medication I was on because it was scrambling my brain. I had real evidence that in those quiet moments, messages were getting through and my body was responding and I was going to do exactly what I saw in my dream. I was going to stand and I was definitely going to walk!

# Kay

Josh told me about the dreams and the messages he was getting. This made me even more determined than ever to get our A-team in to start the recovery process and start healing Josh. Our A-team now consisted of our trusted chiropractor Simon, an extremely talented psychic Paula, our amazing spiritual healer and massage therapist Isabel, and Simon's wonderful reflexologist Jackie.

Many years ago, a friend of mine had a reading with Paula and thought she was amazingly accurate, so I thought I would go along and have one myself. The details she told me were so accurate and precise that it would have been believable that she actually lived through them with me. Over the years, we became friends, and during that time Paula gave Josh readings as well.

He didn't always like what Paula told him, but he knew just how accurate she was, so it was no surprise when Josh was constantly asking me when Paula was coming in. I couldn't help but laugh at that because he had a bit of a love-hate relationship with Paula. Don't get me wrong, he loved her, but he just hated some of things she told him—especially when it came to his girlfriends. If Josh was really keen on one, and Paula told him it wasn't going to last, he got really upset and he didn't want to talk to Paula for a while. As much as he hated to admit it, he knew she always had his best interests at heart.

The main reason I was in agreement with mum to bring in the alternative recovery team was because of the doctors' attitudes. Obviously I had an injury that they had seen before and they classed me as being a C5, C6, C7, T1 complete quadriplegic, and that's where it stopped for them. They performed the surgery, relieved the pressure on the cord and repaired the broken vertebrae, popped in a titanium plate, and everything was done!

And of course, they gave the prognosis that I would most probably never walk again. What they failed to realize was that I wasn't done! And mum wasn't done either. I knew the doctors just weren't going to do anything else for me but the healers mum put together were going to do everything else for me, and it was up to me to work with them to fix and heal myself.

# Kay

I was so afraid for Josh being in the hospital by himself. I knew the nurses were doing all they had to do for him medically, but they couldn't attend to him every minute of the day. The nursing team was fantastic and caring but the ICU ward itself was so old and depressing. It gave me more to fear because I thought he needed all the help he could get, and this hospital looked like it could fall down—it was so depressing.

Australia is a modern, wealthy country and we expect our hospitals to be state of the art, so when you are thrown into the Public Hospital System, we expect our health facilities to be the best! Sadly, the Critical Spinal Unit was well below par, which was disappointing given Josh's injury was so debilitating. We tried to remain positive and upbeat but it was difficult.

Josh was admitted as a private patient because he had the highest hospital insurance cover. Yet, all I could see were these sub-standard surroundings. I couldn't help but wonder how my son was going to progress in surroundings that gave him little confidence and were so old. I certainly had more to worry about than the peeling paint in the ward, but with Josh so critically injured, I had no confidence in the facility itself. This just made me more and more frightened for him.

Josh was unable to eat. He was fed through a tube that was placed down his throat; I found this extremely confrontational, because then I had to deal with the possibility that Josh was going to be bedridden for the rest of his life and they were feeding him in the same manner that he was fed when he was a baby struggling in the Special Care Nursery.

According to the Medical team, I faced the real risk of having a beautiful fit 18-year-old man who was now not much better than a newborn baby.

There were no positive or encouraging words from any of the medical team.

I thought, *How can Josh be protected in this environment?*

I had to fight every emotion to stay positive. It was so hard. There were moments when I felt like disintegrating into tears and just wailing, but I was too scared to do so in fear that I would never stop. I was also acutely aware of staying positive for Josh and everyone else, so I quickly pulled myself together at these times.

One of the skills I learned at Life Mastery was how to change my mood and attitude in a heartbeat. Little did I know I would be exercising this new skill in a way I would have never imagined. I understood now more than ever how important it was to have Josh surrounded by positive people. Keeping his immediate surroundings supportive was achieved by having all Josh's snowboard gear, photographs, and everything that kept Josh focused on his life—the life that he was living and was going to keep living! I wanted above all for Josh to see that we all believed he would get his life back.

We realized he could not be on his own and it was absolutely essential to be with him 24/7. Since I was self-employed, it was really simple—if I didn't work then I wasn't paid, but we managed somehow! If I had to leave the hospital, my sister was there with Josh or our mother stayed. It was difficult because there was so little room where they had Josh set up but we stayed with him probably 20 out of 24 hours of each day, especially in the first week.

Once he was transferred to the Critical Spinal Unit, I knew I had to sleep there with him. I asked for a small bed to be moved next to Josh. The nurses did not allow it and they told me I couldn't sleep there. Not to be outdone, I dragged in on my own—a stained, filthy sofa from the waiting room—and placed it next to Josh's bed. I found the sheets stash and made up the sofa. From then on for the next week, every morning, I dragged the sofa back to the waiting room and brought it back into Josh's room each night. Not once did anyone offer to help me!

I slept in the hospital most nights. I left around 5:00 a.m. to go home for a shower and change of clothes and returned to the hospital just after breakfast. Sleeping next to Josh was totally against the doctors' and nurses' wishes, but I didn't care. My focus

/as only on Josh and no one else. It might sound a bit selfish, but
a our view the hospital was about what you can't do, not what you
can do.

Our rule to the medical team was simply, "If you can't tell us
something positive don't say anything at all!"

There was an incident early on in my admission to hospital that was the
catalyst for me in knowing there was a better and more effective way for
me to recover. One time, the nurses prepared a bath for me so my whole
body could be washed. They placed me in a waterproof bed. The sides
of the bed came up a little so the water didn't go all over the floor. All I
had to cover my private bits was a small towel.

The nurse bathed me by gently hosing me down first. I had one of
these baths before. It was so nice to be bathed. I felt clean after them.
Even though I only felt my shoulders and my armpits getting washed, it
still felt good.

So here I was, in the waterproof bed in the bathroom, and all I had
covering my pelvis area was a small towel. I had nothing else covering
my body. I was bare skinned and totally exposed. I was also still quite wet
from the wash. I had a neck brace on, which was wet from being hosed
down, and it felt heavy and cold around my neck. I wanted to take it off.

Just as the nurse went to get me out of the water and put me onto the
bed, the buzzer went off and she said, "Hang on, I won't be a sec," and
she quickly ran off to attend to something else while she left me in the
bath soaking wet.

An hour passed before she or anyone else came back. I lay in freezing
water for that whole time and I went into shock. I felt my whole body
shut down and I completely freaked out. I still had a collapsed lung from
my accident, and because of that, I couldn't breathe properly. I couldn't
reach the buzzer to notify the nurses, and I couldn't even call out because the feeding tube they had inserted had irritated my vocal cords. I
couldn't even speak, let alone call out to anyone. I was in a lot of distress.
I couldn't believe they could be so negligent and just forget about me.

When they finally realized I wasn't in my room in bed and that they
forgot about me in the bath, they panicked. By the time they reached
me, my whole body was a shivering mess. They got me into bed and they
wrapped me in hot towels straight out from the dryer, and they put space

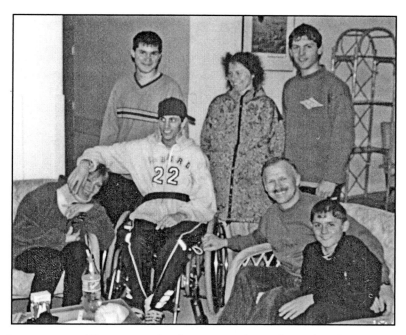

blankets on me. They completely wrapped me from head to toe—all I had was my face showing out of the towels.

Then mum and Paula came into my room.

# Kay

The morning after the accident, I spoke to Paula. She was more than just my psychic healer; she was also my best friend. Like everyone else, she was devastated by Josh's accident. I knew I could count on Paula to help, guide, and support Josh and I through this horror. I had total trust in Paula's psychic healing abilities to help Josh recover and he did too.

She said something extremely important: "You must stay with Josh in the hospital for four to five months. You must be there for him. You cannot trust that he will be okay unless you are with him. If you can't be with him, then Wendy must be there." She went on to say, "By giving Josh that time, you will give him the base for his recovery."

I asked her when she would come in to visit Josh, she simply answered, "When I am ready."

I knew Paula well enough and for long enough by now to understand that she was gathering her energy for what was to become one of her greatest challenges yet, and in my opinion her greatest achievement. Little did we know how important and dramatic her first visit to the hospital to attend Josh would be.

I was not home from the hospital for long when the phone rang. It was Paula.

All she said to me was, "We have to go to the hospital now! Something has happened to Josh, come collect me now."

Every morning, she did her usual healing meditation for Josh by asking for guidance and on this particular morning, she was told to go to the hospital immediately—Josh needed her! I picked Paula up and we sped through the busy Melbourne traffic to get to the hospital. A few days earlier Josh was moved to the Critical Spinal Unit 13 from ICU. Arriving at the hospital, I did my usual trick of dumping the car in any empty space I could find as close to the ward entry as I could get and with Paula and we raced to his ward.

When we reached Josh, he was in a terrible state; he was shivering violently and the nursing staff was piling warm blankets on him. He was so layered and bulked up with the blankets covering him. Josh couldn't speak because they fed him through a tube, which damaged his voice box.

I screamed at a nurse, "What have you done?"

I was so afraid for Josh. My fear for his well-being was elevated to a level no one could imagine. She didn't know where to look, so I repeated myself. She told me that one of the nurses was giving Josh a bath and something had happened, so the nurse was called away and she forgot about him.

Poor Josh couldn't call out due to his damaged throat from the feeding tube, so he lay there freezing and unable to move or call for help until they realized and came back for him an hour later.

While I was berating nurses for their total lack of care of my son, Paula slowly approached Josh and said, "I am just going to sort out this stress you are experiencing."

She walked to his bed and put her fingers on his crown chakra said some calming words, spun the area with her fingers, and said, "Your mum and I are going for a coffee. We'll be back in 10 minutes."

When we returned, Josh was peaceful and relaxed. For the first time in 10 days, he knew there was another way for his recovery—

an alternative—a way that worked. We had a solution! Slowly he began his recovery totally confident he would walk again.

After this experience, there were many days Paula would call me and say, "I have to see Simon today."

On these days, I would call Simon and arrange a coffee meeting for the three of us. Paula often didn't understand the messages she was getting, so she either drew on the back of a napkin what she was being told or just walk Simon through the message.

I remember one such day when she drew around Josh's lower trunk area—just lines that weren't connected. Simon realized it was Josh's meridian lines, so the message Paula received was that we needed to work on Josh's chi energy because he was no longer able to hold onto this energy force in his body. So Simon and Paula discussed a series of adjustments that Simon did to start Josh's body to retain the chi energy.

On the morning that Josh had been left in the bath, the messages came in loud and clear that day and they were telling her that Josh was in trouble.

I had no clue what Paula did to me at the time, but it distracted me enough that I knew that she knew what was going on with me, and I knew I had to trust her. After that, she calmed me down and talked to me.

I had that faith in her. She was on my side and would help me. I know it wasn't anything to do with the hot towels the nurses put on me because they tried that for an hour before mum and Paula came in and it didn't work. And then within five minutes of Paula arriving and doing her thing, I started to feel like myself again.

This frightening episode that I experienced only reaffirmed my belief that I was a prisoner in my own body. It also reaffirmed for me that I was not going to stay like this. I was going to recover, heal, and walk! From then on, mum started bringing in my alternative team one at a time.

Paula was a physic healer. I met Paula years before my accident when mum dragged me along to sit in on one of her readings, which also turned out to be a reading for me. I didn't have a great relationship with Paula. I really couldn't stand her because she told me about accidents I'd have and relationships that wouldn't work and all this life stuff. I didn't like knowing what was going to happen in my future. I was someone that liked to live every day like it was an adventure by not knowing what it was going to bring me.

When I had my accident, I felt like the doctors weren't in my corner. I knew Paula was one person who was in my corner. When she came in to see me, she never promised me I would walk.

She would say, "You know Josh, these are the people I think will help you."

And that's all I needed to hear because I knew the alternative practitioners that came in were supportive and encouraging and wanted to see me achieve my goal to walk. This was so unlike the doctors that gave me no hope and were still trying to make me accept their prognosis that I wouldn't walk, or even be able to get out of bed for that matter.

If any of the doctors just said to me, "Mate, you've done a pretty good job of crushing your spinal cord and breaking your neck and we have done all we can to fix you and at this moment your legs aren't working. But, you never know what improvement you might make," then that would have been enough for me.

That would have been all I needed from them to think that maybe there was some hope—some chance that I could possibly get something

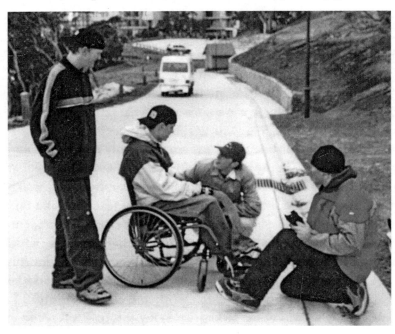

back. I understand that they have a certain duty of care and they have to be careful to not give false hope, but they gave me absolutely no hope. So where was their duty of care for me?

## Kay

> Josh lost nearly one-third of his body weight in the first few weeks after his accident. This was frightening!
>
> Simon's words kept swimming around in my head, "if you don't use it, you'll lose it".
>
> My view was that if Josh couldn't use what was left of his functioning cord, then we would use it for him. The very next morning after Josh was admitted we commenced the massaging of his fingers, hands, toes, and feet using essential oils. It was therapeutic for us all because we felt like we were contributing towards Josh's recovery, even though he couldn't feel the massaging and the stimulation of his fingers and toes. At times he definitely didn't like us doing it, but he understood why we needed to do it.
>
> The doctors and nurses said we were wasting our time doing the massages and that it wouldn't help. We didn't listen and kept doing it.

Isabel came in to see me. She was a spiritual healer, which is a person who uses spirit guides to give her information and help her determine what sort of healing she needed to do for whoever she was working on. Isabel was one of Paula's associate. We hadn't really met before the accident, but we formed a bond straight away and we had this trust in each other. I was happy to have her work on me.

The initial healings she did on me were to align my chakras. She said they needed to be brought back into balance—into my body's energy plane for the recovery process to commence. I always felt so relaxed and calm after her visits when she worked on me.

From just after being transferred to the Critical Ward, Isabel came in weekly for a couple of hours at a time, always later in the night. She continued her visits the whole time I was in hospital and later in rehab.

Most times, she came in with either mum or Paula and we'd did our usual secret healings behind closed curtains.

My body had been broken a lot over the years. I had heaps of injuries and had also been really sick. When I was about 12 years of age, I had a severe staph infection from my horse, which put me in hospital for two weeks. Obviously nothing ever prepared me for spinal cord injury, but I kind of had an idea of what my body could overcome and what was possible to get back.

I made myself think that I had just broken every single bone in my body and I had to repair it. That way, my goal to walk felt more achievable. Because of the times when I woke up from my dreams to find myself sitting up straight in bed combined with some spasms I experienced in my feet and toes, I began to really believe that my movement was coming back.

When I mentioned it to the doctors or nurses, they'd say, "It's just a spasm. That's not your body getting movement back."

I thought to myself, *Hang on, it is my body! So how did these spasms happen?*

I tried to figure out how I could trigger the spasms to work. I thought that if I could get the spasms to work more—even though they were painful and they were completely wrong and they felt bad—it was still movement.

I needed to get my mind clear and stop all the scrambling thoughts that were going on in my brain so that I could focus and begin to make the mind-body connection to get my body responding and moving.

The first thing I did to clear my mind was get off the medication the medical team had me on. I spoke to a couple of nurses and doctors and asked them which pills were the painkillers, because it was obvious that the painkillers weren't working. I felt like I was on fire 24/7 and the messages to my brain were so scrambled that my brain didn't know what information to take in and what to leave out. I was just exhausted all the time.

There was one nurse I kept asking which pills were which. She didn't know why I was asking her, but eventually, she told me which ones were painkillers and which ones weren't. She also told me about the ones I obviously needed to take to survive, such as the blood thinners so I didn't get blood clots.

Once I knew which were the painkillers, I slid them straight off the side of the bed or the table into the bin. I even got my mates to throw them into the bin. They all thought I was mad!

Everyone told me, "You won't survive the first week because there's no way you can deal with this pain."

And I said, "Well this is not working. You are giving me 40 tablets each day, and none of the pain is subsiding, so I'd rather be off them."

In the first week, after being transferred to the Acute Ward, I was completely off all painkillers.

Once I was off those, I had more clarity within my brain, and I thought, *Okay, now I'll use this clarity to work out how to connect my brain to my feet.*

Even though I couldn't feel my legs, I would lay there in bed and they would be straight, but they felt like they were hanging off the end of the bed.

So I just visualized that my legs were straight and I kept telling my brain, *My legs are straight, my legs are straight.*

It took me weeks, but after a while, my brain started figuring out that it shouldn't listen to the mixed messages. I still experienced a lot of involuntary feeling and phantom pain. I could describe it like when someone is an amputee and they say they feel the leg is still there but it's not. It's like that, but obviously the difference is my legs are actually still there, but my brain can't feel them at all.

Once I started getting off the painkillers and connecting my brain to my body and doing the visualization, it really started to work and I began to feel some sensation, which was in my legs.

I kept the whole process simple. I kept dumbing it down. I definitely didn't research anything about my condition or what progress I could expect or not expect. I wasn't interested in finding out what I wasn't meant to have, because as soon as I did know or find out what I wasn't meant to have, then it would be stuck in my head.

It was like the saying, "What you don't know can't hurt you".

I had to be very mindful of any information or messages that I was exposed to because once that message was in my head, it would have stayed there. Any information I knew about my condition was always going to be in the back of my mind, like when I would go to do something like try to stand or even take a step, there was a message inside my head that would say, *Oh no, you can't, because it's your injury and you can't do it.*

From there, I worked with my psychic healer Paula who taught me visualization techniques to connect my brain to my body. Isabel taught me meditation techniques as well. These techniques allowed me to quiet my mind and stop all the scrambling messages so I could get clear and focus.

At the same time, my body was becoming cleared of blockages and stagnant energy. Between Paula and Isabel, some very powerful healing was happening.

It worked for me; it might not be someone else's way of doing things, and it might not work for everybody else, but it worked for me.

# Chapter 3 – Part 2

# When No Hope is Given

## I had my A-team. Now we were going to kick goals.

### Kay

With the alternative part of Josh's healing going along very well, Paula continued to meditate to receive the road map to Josh's recovery by utilizing her unique skills. We continued to draw the curtains around Josh's bed. The nurses seemed to accept our need for privacy and didn't question it. All visitors were told to close the curtains whenever they visited, so at night when our work was being done, so no one questioned us.

Josh's father felt Josh should bond with his fellow injured patients in the ward. This was something I really dissuaded Josh from doing. I didn't want him to hear the hardships, battles, and frustrations that others were going through. I also didn't want Josh to take on their fears and frustrations. We were always pleasant and polite to everyone else in the ward, but my only concern was Josh, and it was enough for us to focus just on his issues. I found the whole Acute Spinal Ward experience extremely negative and distressingly sad with no great healing or recovery objective. The message from the medical team was always, without fail, acceptance of the prognosis. This was totally the opposite message of what we presented and instilled into Josh. We slowly gained evidence that our non-traditional approach was working.

It's one thing to have gone through my accident, but situations like the one when I was forgotten and left in a bath made me realize just how vulnerable I was in the hospital system when I was so dangerously injured. I should have always felt safe, but I was constantly scared shitless wondering what and when something else would happen. I didn't expect things to go wrong in a place where I should have been the most protected and supported—especially when I was by myself in my most injured and vulnerable state. Unfortunately, I experienced that lack of care a few more times with different incidents while I was in hospital.

I was just trying to survive, let alone deal with all these extra stressful situations that continually happened. I always used those experiences to keep me strong, focused, and determined to achieve my goal to walk.

The massaging my friends and family did on me, combined with the chakra clearing and energy bodywork Isabel did, was all working well. Even though I felt more confident in getting movement back, I was never satisfied with my progress, so I started intensifying the visualization techniques that Paula taught me.

One time when I was lying in bed, I had this message that I was going to move my feet. I remembered there was a chart—a male human body anatomy chart that hung on the wall in the hospital hall—so I asked a nurse if she would please bring it to me and position it next to my bed so I could look at it and study it. I could then understand how all the muscles, ligaments, and tendons worked and connected throughout my body. I thought I had nothing to lose by giving it a go. So, I closed my eyes and visualized the view through an imaginary video camera moving from my eyes through my body, going down my legs, right to where my toes were, and where the little tendons were.

Then, I pretended I was a puppeteer. Just like a puppeteer pulls on the strings to make his puppets move, I visualized that I pulled on the ligaments and tendons. I did this puppeteer visualization technique for hours. After about two days of continually doing this visualization, my big toe kicked—it moved! I nearly cried with excitement. It was tough to keep focused and not give up but I knew I had to be relentless in my goal and not give in. I wasn't going anywhere so I had to give myself every chance and opportunity. I didn't know if it was going to work but I had to keep focused.

I hadn't seen my toe move in nearly two weeks, and I thought, *Hang on—is that me making my toe move or is it the spasms?*

So I repeated the visualization and it worked again! I had moved my big toe on my own. I was so excited to the point of tears again. It sounds weird, but I couldn't remember how to move my toes because it wasn't a natural movement for me at that recovery stage, so I had to think of things that weren't natural. I remembered the feeling of when I put my feet in grass or in sand and I would grip it with my toes. That's what I pretended to do. I had to visualize the movement and see it in my mind because I couldn't feel if it was working.

The first moment I saw my big toe twitch, I got so excited that I wanted to show my nurse what I managed to do.

When she came in, I said, "Check this out," and I showed her that I was able to move my big toe.

This small movement became my new party trick. I showed off for a few weeks. I knew that once I could move my big toe, I would just work all the way back and get movement and sensation happening throughout my whole body.

From that moment on, I kept practicing my visualization every minute, because now that I had some movement back, I wasn't going to lose it. When I woke up every morning I was excited to see what movement I would get back next. When people came in to see me, I got them to pull the sheet off my foot and I showed them what bit of my body was waking up again. And that's how I had to look at it—nothing was paralyzed, but it was just asleep and I never let my mind think any different. When I got new movements back, it reassured me that it was possible to get even more and that motivated me every day.

Every time some new movement came back, in my mind I was like, *Agh, sweet, a bit more of my body has decided to join us!*

The nurses were fine watching me perform my little twitch show, and the doctors were like, "Oh yeah well, that's just probably an involuntary movement. Most people get that and you'll most probably lose it."

Never once did the doctors say, "That's awesome Josh, that's a sign that you might get something back."

My biggest hospital support group was the turners.

Those guys got so pumped for me and said, " Man, this is awesome, we hardly ever see stuff like this."

# Kay

As Paula received her messages, she introduced Josh to more and more ways for him to gain more recovery. Her first project was to teach Josh visualization techniques. She taught him to visualize his body waking up and being healed and at the same time, to visualize the pain leaving his body. Visualization is an extremely difficult skill to master. It required total concentration but Josh became expert at it very quickly. With all the negativity around him, he craved anything that was positive. Visualizing the pain leaving his body allowed him to get off the morphine, which the medical team really pushed on him. The medical team fought us every step of the way on what Josh's medication should be and the amount of medication they should have him on. We questioned them on the necessity of one drug or another, or anything that we weren't convinced was really necessary to his recovery. We told them to remove those from his medicine regime. Josh was convinced that his brain was scrambled because of all the medication, so in order to be able to meditate, and more importantly, visualize, he needed to his head to be clear.

Josh decided the first body part that he work on was going to be his big toe on his left foot. There were two reasons that he chose this part:

1.  Josh was left sided. He wrote with his left hand, he snowboarded with his left foot forward, he kicked a ball with his left foot, and he did everything left.
2.  The toes were the furthest part of the body from the point of injury, so there were more muscles, tendons and ligaments to get passed to connect to. So in Josh's theory, if he could connect and get movement out of his extremities, then he could get movement anywhere in his body.

When Josh successfully moved his big toe through the visualization technique, we were all jubilant! I guess that was another one of those moments that we knew anything was possible, and more importantly, so did Josh! Paula continually worked with Josh to perfect his visualization skills. Josh found it hard to sleep, so he continued to take medication for this.

Paula was adamant that he needed to have his body as pure as possible, so Josh slowly weaned himself off the sleeping tablets.

He had to eat clean and well and have no alcohol in his body. He had to be as pure as possible and because Josh began to see the results, he listened to her and embraced everything she said.

Another healing therapy that worked very well on Josh was the use of crystals. The crystals concentrated on all areas of Josh's body—not just the areas that were impacted. Paula came into the hospital once or twice a week for a couple of hours to work with Josh, whether it was with her crystals, or enhancing his visualization skills, or just encouraging him with his recovery.

My body began to respond to all the therapies and techniques I learned and applied every day. I slowly had my sensation and movement back because I was diligent on the fact that we had the alternative therapists in straight away and I started applying all their techniques immediately from their first visits.

I remember one day a nurse came in to roll me onto my stomach to give my back a bit of relief.

She said to me, "Do you reckon you could squeeze your bum?"

In those early days after my accident, I was naked for most of the time because I couldn't have any elastic or anything restrictive around my body since I had very poor circulation. She rolled me over and my butt was just hanging up in the air and she got me to try to squeeze my butt cheeks. She pinched the top part of my bum or the top part of my thigh and then my leg spasmed.

I said, "I felt that!"

And from then on I learned how to clench my butt cheeks. When I was rolled over, I saw all these nurses standing at the doorway of my room looking at me and giving each other high fives. That was probably one of the only times the medical staff gave me encouragement.

It got me thinking about other spinal cord injured people who could possibly move parts of their body but they didn't know how to connect to it and get that response. So from then, on I got people to pinch different parts of my legs and body to try to connect and get movement and sensation into that particular area.

## Kay

Very early in the injury, Paula involved our third key recovery person Isabel. She was a spiritual healer and massage therapist who always worked with spirit. The universe was her assistant. Her initial role was to realign Josh's chakras, which according to Isabel, were intact but all over the place. Her work was meticulous. I brought her into the acute spinal unit late at night with Paula. We did our usual "privacy please" closing of the curtains around Josh's bed and she began her amazing work. Isabel usually worked on Josh for two hours at a time once a week. Her goals were to keep the energy flowing through Josh's body and realign his chakras, which were being the life force of the internal body.

Sitting with these two remarkable women was always a privilege because they were so dedicated to getting Josh back on his feet, and the energy around the healing was phenomenal. Josh always felt Isabel working on him, even though in these early parts of his journey he was still completely paralyzed. Balancing and realigning Josh's chakras reduced his stress. It had a calming effect on him and he started to feel a lot better and more connected with his broken body. Josh gained confidence everyday that our radical approach to his recovery was the right way to go. Josh regarded Isabel as the best who ever worked on him.

We were always grateful to them for their work. Personally, I believe their commitment and early involvement set Josh up for his ongoing recovery.

When my chiropractor Simon came in, he never did any manipulation movements on me.

What he said was, "Okay, these nerves represent this. If you massage this, then the messages will become clearer."

He never structurally adjusted me in any way. He simply pushed his fingers very lightly on the different pressure points of my body. I felt it sometimes. I felt just a hint of something. Then he used this other hand-held instrument. It had a handle with a wheel with spurs on its edges and he rolled it on different spots of my body: arms, legs, and torso. Sometimes, he gently used it on my face. My face was the only place I had 100% sensation. I felt what the contact sensation actually felt like. Knowing how it felt, I visualized it on the other areas of my body.

Sometimes Simon rolled the spurs on my body and I didn't feel a thing, but then it hit a certain spot and I had a patch of sensation. It wasn't pain—it was just a contact feeling but we kept at it and after a time, different feelings came back.

Not everyone realizes how many different sensations we have. There's light touch, hard touch, pain, hot, and cold, so my body was like a patchwork quilt. There was the odd spot here and there that responded and we never gave up on it.

Every time my stepbrother Andrew came in he gave me nipple cripples. I didn't ever feel it, even when he twisted them so far that they almost snapped off.

Then one day when he did it, my reaction was, "Argh, that hurt!"

He said, "What? Did you feel that?"

And I realized I did indeed feel it.

Then we had a big celebration and he said, "Yep, I told you I'd get your nipples working!"

That's how we did things. We woke up my body very simply.

Later on, when I made a bit more of a recovery, I asked Andrew if he would shave under my chin because the hair had grown and it was really uncomfortable and irritating. The hair kept rubbing up against the neck brace and I could feel the whole area rash up. It took me about half an hour to convince Andrew to shave me right then and there. He finally agreed and pulled the curtains around for privacy. He loosened the neck brace I was wearing from the front, so he could get to the chin hair.

We got stuck into this conversation about his surgery he had the past week. He was involved in a bike accident and got hurt quite badly. He actually ended up having dual knee reconstructions. We talked away and got lost in the conversation and because his legs didn't work properly since they were still healing from his surgery, he repositioned himself to get closer to me to enable him to keep shaving me. Without thinking, he grabbed my face and twisted my head to the side. I heard a crack in my neck. I just absolutely shit myself and he absolutely shit himself.

He went completely white and dropped the razor and I said to him, "What the fuck did you just do to me?"

He just said, "Oh no, what the fuck have I done?"

I said, "Well, move my head back," and he grabbed my chin and went to put my neck brace on me and I said, "What the hell are you doing? Finish shaving my face!"

So he quickly finished the shave, put the neck brace back on me, and then we buzzed the nurse.

She came in and asked what was wrong and I told her I sneezed and I heard my neck crack. As a precaution, they took me to get MRIs done and thankfully there was no sign of damage. My neck was fine.

Nothing cracked that wasn't meant to crack, and after that, I thought, *Well if my neck went through that, theoretically I should be able to take the neck brace off at the front and move my head around.*

I previously had this vision of when the doctors finally took the neck brace off that my head was going to fall off my shoulders, but it didn't happen. After this experience, I gained confidence and was a bit cocky I suppose. I decided to start and take the brace off and let my neck strengthen on its own.

I convinced my mates that the nurses said it was fine if they unstrapped the front of the neck brace, but left the back on, just to let my neck breathe. My mates used to unstrap the front and ever so lightly I moved my head backwards and forwards and up and down, just to keep that muscle memory and improve my neck strength. Whether it helped or not, I don't know. All I know is that it felt great to take the neck brace off after seven weeks and when I took it off, I didn't feel like my head was going to fall off my shoulders.

That was another turning point. I knew I had to do whatever I could do that I thought was possible and not think about what I was told was impossible. I wasn't meant to be in a wheelchair, but guess what? My first goal was to get into a wheelchair. It wasn't long before the day came and I did exactly that—get into a wheelchair. The nurses got me out of bed and dressed me. It felt great after practically being naked for three weeks. It was really exciting for me because it was the first time I was out of the bed in about three weeks. To get me into the wheelchair wasn't an easy process. After dressing me, the nurses put the harness under me and attached the harness to a mini crane that lifted me out of bed and slowly lowered me into the wheelchair. This whole process took about 35 minutes.

As they sat me in the wheelchair and pulled the harness out from underneath me, I shat my pants. My body had been lying down and was immobile in one spot for so long that once I was sat upright, I just exited everything I had in my bowels.

It broke my heart and I thought, *Look what am I going through. Is this what it is going to be like for the rest of my life?*

There I was, sitting in my own shit.

Immediately, I went through a list in my mind of all the times this would happen and I repeated over and over in my head, *Is this what it's going to be for the rest of my life?*

It brought all the challenges of going to the toilet back into my mind. In the very beginning of being in hospital, if I needed to pee, I had a bag hanging off the side of the bed, with a tube hanging out that went all the way into my bladder. If I had to poo, the nurse physically stuck a suppository up my butt because I had no movement. Then, I had to poo in my bed. The nurse rolled me over and I lay on my side and I would poo into a blue cloth thing and after I finished, they used that same cloth to wipe me up from behind. It was an extremely demeaning experience.

To get my stools working, they used to stick their finger up my butt. One nurse did it once, and she was so rough and it was just so bad, and I wondered if this was what my life was going to be like. This is the stuff that no one talks about. Most people think that when someone breaks their neck it's just their legs that won't work. Well, that's nothing compared to everything else you go through. It's demeaning, and the worst thing is that you don't have any other option and you have to do it this way.

When people see someone in a wheelchair, it's quite common to think that what they are seeing is someone who just can't walk. That's only the surface. There is so much more that the person in the chair goes through. Bladder and bowel functions are the two main concerns let alone all the other stuff that needs to be dealt with on a daily basis. I honestly feel they are the two biggest issues. Sometimes, they are even more of a concern than not being able to use your legs. The body and its functions become so unpredictable and every situation is different every day. There is so much that just can't be controlled. Every spinal cord injury case is different. Not one person has the same issue as another.

I was just an 18-year-old kid. Prior to the accident, I was totally independent. I lived on my own and lived the dream, so this was extremely tough on me.

And then I dropped everything that was in my bowels all over my clothes, the chair, and myself. My joy and excitement of finally getting out of bed turned into absolute horror. The nurses put me back into bed and they cleaned me up. I was really scared to get back in the chair again because I didn't want to shit myself again.

I started to think, *If I'm scared now, then tomorrow I'm going to be scared as well, and again the next day.*

I knew I had to just get over it or I would be too scared to do anything, so after cleaning me up and dressing me, I was once more lowered into the wheelchair and this time, I was fine. I didn't shit myself!

It was good to finally be up and out of bed.

I was told later that it was quite normal for this to happen the first time someone with a cord injury gets out of bed. I just wished they warned me. I could have mentally prepared myself for it. The problem with this injury was that there was so much to learn and it seemed I always learned the hard way.

I sat in the chair and looked at people front on instead of having them look down on me lying flat. That was another little milestone for me and I celebrated it. I knew I had to celebrate every little accomplishment along the way. If I didn't appreciate or feel grateful for what I had, then I would forget about how far I came or lose sight of what my plan and goals were. So I always made sure I celebrated everything, big and small.

Initially, I didn't want to ever use a wheelchair. I wanted to just get out of bed and walk, but then I realized that using the chair was the only way of getting some independence. In time, I knew the wheelchair was going to be my legs, so getting into the wheelchair was as good as standing.

Being in the chair changed my world. I could look at people, I could sit up and eat food without lying down, and I was mobile! It was those mini milestones that kept me focused on my overall goal to walk again. At first, I couldn't push the wheelchair myself because I didn't have enough movement and strength in my arms and hands to power it on my own, so I was pushed around.

It took me a few more weeks and I started to let my hands just run along the tops of the wheels so I could feel the movement of them. I had special gloves with grips but I hated them. I thought they looked really shitty so I had my motorbike gloves brought in. I didn't have enough strength to pull the gloves on myself, so my friends put them on me. The gloves had grips on the palms, so I used to go around in the chair and just grip at the wheels. Sometimes it was a bit sketchy when I couldn't stop but it felt great to be able to move on my own.

I kept working at getting stronger in the chair every day. I was about six weeks in from when I first had the surgery on my neck. I was stable and spent more of my day in the chair than in bed, so the time came up to transfer to the rehabilitation centre to further my recovery. I was really excited and I thought it was going to be great because it was supposedly the best rehab centre in our state and I had heard all about it.

I thought that they would help me walk, get my arms and legs moving, and start me getting my independence back.

I was transferred across from the hospital to the rehab centre by ambulance. My dad drove over from his house to the centre and met me at the entrance just as I arrived. During my last week in hospital, I had these dreams about riding Harleys again—that I had my life back, and another dream was that I was going to walk out of rehab.

I had no clue what the rehab centre looked like but I kept having this dream of sliding doors and I was walking out on crutches. It was a lot to think about but it was so believable in my mind that I let myself think that it was really going to happen and I was going to make sure it was nothing less than that.

When we pulled up in the ambulance, I saw what the centre looked like. It was exactly like it was in my dream, so I thought for a second that it wasn't a dream and that that maybe I had seen a future event in my mind and I was having a déjà vu experience.

I was on the stretcher and as the stretcher has come out of the ambulance, before it got to the sliding doors I said to my dad, "I'm going to walk out of these doors before my nineteenth birthday."

Dad said, "Well mate, you've got to have your goals, but just don't put too much pressure on yourself."

It was a fair comment from dad given that my birthday was only three and a half months away. For me, it didn't feel like a lot of pressure, but it did to everyone else because at that time I wasn't even anywhere near standing.

When I was wheeled into the admissions centre, they sat down with me and went through their program. They explained what they were going to do, how they were going to help me, and about the physiotherapists, the occupational therapist, and all about their programs. It was exciting because I thought this was where I was going to get my life back again and it was all going to start that day.

With all the visualization I did and the massages I had, I began to get a bit more movement in my arms and hands. I could almost shake hands with someone with my right hand, and with my left hand I could push the wheelchair, so in my eyes that was enough to start building upon.

I still wasn't able to feed myself. I couldn't cut my food because I couldn't put pressure on the fork or cut meat with a knife, and I wasn't able to hold a glass to drink from, so everyone still had to feed me and give me drinks. I didn't have any coordination with that, but it was only something I had to relearn. The main thing was that I was out of hospital and in the rehab centre, and I was excited to be there.

I didn't train for the first week because I had a bladder infection. I caught it while I was in hospital from the catheter. I couldn't urinate properly and had a catheter inserted, which was attached to an external bag placed on my leg. The whole catheter-bag set up wasn't working properly for me so I ended up with a bladder infection. So I spent the first week getting used to my new surroundings and familiarizing myself with the layout of the building and the staff who worked with me. I couldn't wait to start the training programs. I felt like I would train well because my lungs had become stronger over the time I was in hospital and I didn't run out of breath anymore.

When I was in hospital, I had to do a breath test where I blew into a tube and tried to get all four balls to float to the top. They had me do this test a few times a day every single day. I just thought it was routine. I didn't realize that I could have died in the first weeks because I could barely get one ball to rise, let alone four balls up in the air. After about two or three weeks, I was able to get all four balls raised.

After my first week in the centre, they said I could start the rehab program. In my mind I planned to do three or four hours of training per day. I had my first meeting with my rehab team and they did nothing! They just laid me on the bed and had me move my arms around.

They didn't even touch my legs and I thought, *What's going on? Aren't I meant to do all this stuff with my legs?*

I asked the physiotherapist, "When are we going to do rehab with my legs?"

And they said, "Look, we'll stretch them out for you but there's no real use doing anything with your legs because you're never going to walk again."

If I could have kicked them, I would have booted the shit out of them. I was so pissed!

I thought, *This is fucking rehab! I've been told this is the best rehab in Victoria and one of the best in Australia, and their theory is that just because this is what I've been told, this is all I'm going to get?*

I wasn't off to a good start and that place obviously wasn't going to help me recover the way I thought, hoped, and planned. What the fuck was I going to do now? I felt totally let down by the system—I was devastated! I quickly became a problem patient there because I believed I was going to get better.

I wanted to do the work and the training to recover as much as possible, but they had the same narrow-minded attitude as the doctors in the hospital had, which was, "You probably won't walk again Josh," "you're a quadriplegic Josh," "you might get enough movement back to sit in a wheelchair, but that's about it," and all the rest of verbal shit they kept repeating to me.

They even sent me to see the psychologist at the rehab centre because they didn't think I dealt with my accident since I always smiled.

I said to the psychologist, "The reason why I'm smiling is because I see someone worse off every single day getting around in a wheelchair by their chin, using their chin to move and steer the electric chair and they smile every day, so who am I to whinge about the situation I'm in?"

I don't know if they understood what I meant but I didn't care, and this was exactly how I looked at my situation. It was my fault that I had this accident. I wasn't thrown out of a car. It wasn't someone else's fault because no one else hurt me. It was my fault, so I had no right to feel sorry for myself.

I played along with the physiotherapist and occupational therapist programs, knowing full well that they weren't interested in helping me achieve my goal to walk, but I was happy to get any time with them and get any sort of stimulus training. I went along to rehab and they stretched my legs out, but never really did anything else with my legs. The OT (occupational therapist) used putty on my hands to do strength tests and to see if I could squeeze it or mould it into different shapes. I used lifting blocks to learn how to lift up blocks, and place the square into the square one and the round into the round one. I never played Jenga because I found it difficult to try to get the wooden blocks to balance on top of each other and I kept knocking them over. I felt like I went back to being a little kid. I went back to being like a baby as I had to learn balance and coordination skills all over again. It was basically about trying different ways to get my body to remember.

Dingo brought in a PlayStation and he said, "This should help your hands."

I couldn't even hold the controls at that stage.

I tried playing a game and I couldn't even do it, and I thought, *only seven weeks ago before I had my accident, I played this same PlayStation game and I was fine.*

Dingo kept saying, "Just keep doing it mate, you'll get it."

I just kept trying, and after a few weeks I started getting dexterity in my fingers and it gave me confidence to start doing other things with my hands. I also found that using my mobile to learn how to punch in the numbers allowed me to keep in touch with family and friends. It was good motivation to get my fingers working. Mum never complained about my mobile bills, even though some months they were over $1,000. She was just happy that I could call, and that I was regaining more independence.

I wanted to eat properly, so they gave me a knife and fork with special handles and I said to them, "I'm going to starve myself before I use that stuff."

So I made myself learn how to hold onto regular cutlery; at first I couldn't even hold onto them. I placed the fork in my hand and I pushed my fingers to close around the fork with my other hand until it felt tight and then I just tried my hardest to hold the grip. After a few weeks, I learned to hold a fork and put it in my mouth. That was just enough to be able to feed myself. I expected everything to come back—all my skills and coordination—and that's how I made sure I made progress. I kept thinking that it was just going to be like that.

When I first went to rehab, I shared a room with someone else. One thing about people with a spinal cord injury is that they are never comfortable, so when they get ready to go to sleep, 99 percent of spinal cord injury people don't ever sleep properly. If they try to go to sleep and the other bloke is awake in the room, then they never get any rest. Because of this, I knew I had to get into my own room.

I said to the nurses, "What do I have to do to get out of this room cause I'm so sick of sharing it with someone. I want my own room."

They said, "Oh no, it will take you two months to learn how to be independent enough to have your own room. You have to be able to do your own bowel program, you have to be able to do your own exchange into the wheelchair and into bed, and you have to..." The list went on.

I said, "Give me a laundry list of what I have to do and I'll be able to do it by the end of the week."

One of the nurses I, who got along with, wrote out a list of what I needed to do and I said to her, "Come back in a week and I'll be doing it."

She said, "Josh, it's impossible, you're not even doing two of those things."

And I said, "Trust me, I'm sick of nurses sticking their fingers up my butt and I'm sick of hearing people snore and scream out in pain. I'm sick of not having my own independence or my own room. I'm sick of being like this, so trust me, this is what I'm going to do."

This was my motivation. In my mind, I didn't have a clue how I was going to do it, but once I had it in my mind that I was going to do it, there was no changing it.

So for the next week I practiced everything and learned how to use the catheter on my own, which took ages. I was in the bathroom for about 15 minutes but I didn't care because I independently did it on my own. I learned how to move in bed, grab onto my dead-weight legs, fight through the spasms, and get my legs close enough to my body so I could put my socks on. I learned how to do some of the most basic of things like how to brush my teeth again. This was all the stuff I took for granted not even eight weeks ago.

Before my accident, I jumped out of bed, stood up, got dressed, bent down, picked my shoes up off the floor, balanced on one leg while I put on each shoe, walked to the bathroom, had a pee, brushed my teeth, walked into the kitchen, grabbed all the food from the fridge in both hands, and did all this within 15 minutes.

Now it took me 20 minutes to just finally get my leg close enough to attempt to put my socks on and it wasn't just my legs I had to fight, but I also had zero core strength or arm strength, so I got tired of fighting everything. Nothing was easy, but I wouldn't let anything beat me. I could have given up and had the nurse or whoever was in the room do it for me. I could have sat back and been less stressed, but I didn't let that happen. I wanted my independence and freedom. I wanted to feel like I was getting a bit of my life back even if it was a simple thing that we all take for granted like putting socks on in the morning.

At the end of that week, I said, "Alright, I'm ready to do it!"

And they said, "Okay well it's going to take three weeks for an assessor to come through and assess you."

I was so pissed off, and I said, "That's bullshit! You can do it—you can assess me yourself and you can see what I've done."

It took about four or five days, and by the end of the week they said, "Okay, we can move you into your own room."

This still took another week, but finally I went into my own room. My friend lent me a small bar fridge; we managed to stock it full with Coca-Cola and fruit juices. Mum brought in my favourite snacks—salt and vinegar chips and chocolate teddy bear biscuits. I even had my television and could now watch my favourite shows. In my room, I also had some of my personal stuff like my snowboard and motorbike gear. We set it all up exactly how I wanted it. The more my living environment resembled a space that I was comfortable in and felt was more uplifting and distant from the hospital and rehab living environments, the better it was for me to cope on a daily basis. It was exactly what my mind needed. It was my escape. I needed to feel like I was living in an apartment where I could escape everyone else's issues. It was also so much easier for my family and friends to visit me and be relaxed.

# Kay

Once Josh was moved to rehab, we fought for a private room. We had no TAC (Transport Accident Charge Insurance), so it was difficult for us to obtain this private room. Most of the people suffering with spinal cord injuries had them through road accidents, so their costs were covered through TAC. However, we relied upon Medicare insurance, so the hospital didn't receive as much income for people like Josh, but we were determined and we eventually won the battle for the private room.

From the start of Josh's admittance to rehab, we noticed that the TAC patients seemed to get more attention from the staff because the TAC paid for their treatment.

The bonus for Josh was that he was finally in his own room with a double bed, which gave him more room to roll around in and get out of. We brought in his bedding from home along with a television, his video games, and a small refrigerator. We dressed and furnished it to have it resemble Josh's home environment as close as possible. This kept us focused on Josh's future instead of dwelling on the sadness of his injury. We still cooked all of Josh's meals except for breakfast. I also organized and set up accounts at some local restaurants so Josh could order what he liked without worrying. Hospital food left a lot to be desired. Frankly, we couldn't have fed the food in rehab to our dogs because it was so bad! Between our home cooking and the quality restaurant food, Josh received nutrients from the balanced variety of food. It was one less thing for me to worry about. He started to gain some of the weight he lost and looked healthier.

Once Josh was in rehab, my fears heightened—especially at night. The rehab centre consisted of two wings at opposite sides of a huge reception area. It was modern in design; there were roughly 28 rooms. Initially, what I feared most was if a fire broke out in the building. At night, there were four nurses on duty at most and usually not even that many, so in the event of a fire, how could they possibly get almost 40 injured people out of the building safely?

On the first day Josh was there, I asked them about the procedure in the case of a fire. I was advised that in the event of one, hospital staff would come down and bring everyone out. I argued the point that with a central stairway, this would be difficult, especially for Josh, so I decided to stay with him until at least 2 a.m. every night and sometimes later. At that stage, he was still quite weak and only just transferring to his chair, so nothing was ever achieved in a hurry.

After a certain time, the facility was locked down, so every night or early morning when I finally left, I had to track down the security guard to let me out. Naturally they weren't happy with me, but frankly I didn't care because my concerns were always for Josh's safety and well-being.

Once Josh was able to transfer to a wheelchair safely and quickly, and he regained more stable movement and mobility, I cut back my hours slightly, leaving most nights about 1 a.m.

Mum, my family, and my friends brought in photos of me doing action sports or movements I did. We put them all around the room so I had the visual of my old life as I lived it prior to the accident. I made sure that my mind never saw anything less than what was in those photos.

We completely decked out the room with photos, pictures, and posters. I had my television and a fridge so when my mates came over, they could have a cold drink. I had everything set up as if I lived in an apartment because that's what I saw when I woke up. I thought the more my brain didn't think I was injured or the more I felt like I was not in a hospital-type environment, then the better I was going to get.

It started working! I learned to trick my mind so well, that if I did it properly and often enough, I started to believe this was my reality. I obviously knew I was in rehab, but I kept chipping away and doing my own thing in my own room and showed myself I was getting better and stronger everyday. I can't stress enough how much I visualized in my room. I did it so intensively that it wore me out.

Then one day, I woke up and I thought, *This is the day I'm going to stand—I had that message in my head.*

When my physiotherapist came in to see me that morning, I said to her, "I'm so excited, I'm going to stand today."

She said, "Josh you need to stop doing this and letting yourself down. You're never going to walk again."

I said, "The only reason I'm letting myself down is because you guys won't let me do what I want to do."

Yet again, we were back on the same old argument.

I butted heads with her for a whole hour and then after all that time arguing, she finally gave up and said, "Alright, fine, let's try it."

After that hour spent arguing my point and using all that energy to get my point across, I was tired and pissed off. Still, they were going to let me try and stand. One physiotherapist held my knees and ankles while the other one sat behind me. They had me between two beds. They were physio beds so they were quite hard and there was a little gap in between them. They placed my legs over the side of one of the beds and then one physiotherapist lifted me up. The other held my legs to the floor as if I was standing. I was wobbly and I kept falling over and then I collapsed. I tried three times but I couldn't stand up. I was so angry and the anger got to me, so I left the physio room to go back to my own room.

The physiotherapists wasted no time in saying to me, "Told you so!"

Later that same morning, Lammo's dad came in to see me. I told him what happened earlier that day. He could tell in my voice that I was still really pissed off.

He said to me, "Josh, you've got to let this anger go—you've got to. You learn from what you've done."

He went over everything that I did and achieved so far in my progress.

I said, "Yeah I know I've been through all that, but I'm just pissed off!"

He said, "Get over it! You've got to stop being pissed off."

Having him tell me to get over it and the way he said it flicked a switch on inside my brain. No one said that to me before, especially in that manner. It made me think that I had to do just that—that I had to get over it and keep moving forward with my progress.

He stayed for a bit longer and then he left to go get lunch. I went back to the rehab gym to do some training and I found that I could hold onto some weights. They were only about half a kilogram, but I could hold them. I got all my anger out in that training session. I swore at myself and talked to myself because there was no one else in the room.

As I rolled out of the gym, I saw the parallel bars. I rolled up to them and I visualized how to stand. At that moment, I couldn't remember how to stand even though it was such a natural thing to do. It became unnatural and I lost all my coordination and ability to do everything I knew how to do before. That's why mentally it felt like I went right back to early childhood, because I had to learn how to do everything all over again.

I took a minute and thought, *What is it like to stand? I need to visualize this movement!*

I thought that if I could associate standing with something similar that I did recently before my accident, then in my brain it would create the same pattern of movement.

I started to think of my motor cross bike when I went through the bumps and I was on the pegs, and I was going up and down. I visualized that feeling, which was an unnatural feeling. On a motor cross bike, when a rider goes to jump, they do an action called preload. They use their body weight to push down on the pegs of the bike and then they lift up so they get that spring-up action. I just felt that in my mind. The same goes for the action with a snowboard; when a snowboarder sits on the ground or has the snowboard placed on the ground with their feet strapped onto the board, they then need that push down and have the spring-up movement to lift the board off the ground. It's an unnatural movement because legs and feet can't move as easily.

I integrated that movement into my mind and said to myself, *Remember how to stand because you've got to remember which muscles to switch on and the sequence of their movement.*

I grabbed my legs and placed them out of the chair so they just touched the floor and as I held the bars I tried to pull myself up. I visualized the preload action in my mind, and I saw myself do that action just like I used to do on my motor cross bike or on my snowboard and I just pushed my body. I sat out of the chair about four inches, then I fell back into it.

I got really angry again, so I said to myself, "Just relax."

I tried it again and fell back in the chair again but I just kept at it.

I kept visualizing the action and I said to myself, "Just breathe and think about what you're doing. Shut the anger down and stop making it so hard on yourself."

And then it worked! I tried one more time and I stood! My hips were so loose and my back had not had that much feeling in a long time. It felt like my arse was going to fall from my legs and I felt like my spine went *click, click, click, click.* It just unlocked so much stiffness and tension that it was unbelievable. My hips felt really flexible. I felt like Elvis Presley standing there with my hips going.

Then I thought, *Make out like you've got your feet in concrete and you're stuck in concrete,* so I just kept visualizing that.

My legs started to spasm and they went everywhere. They were trying to jump out from underneath me.

I just kept thinking, *Focus and breathe.*

I tried to breathe the spasm out and breathe through a calm energy. And then I stood there.

I thought, *I can let go.*

And I did! I let go! I was a bit wobbly in the hips, but I stood there without touching anything.

Of course, me being me, I wasn't going to just stop there so I thought, *Let's take it to the next level,* and I dragged my legs to the end of the parallel bars and I realized, *Shit! How do I get back to my wheelchair?*

To this day I still don't know how I got back but I did—I got back in my wheelchair and I went straight to my physiotherapist to tell her. I wheeled into her office.

She was sitting there eating her lunch, and I said, "Come here, come, come watch this."

She said, "What? I'm having lunch."

And I said, "I know you're having lunch, but you said I'd never move my legs again and I'd never walk again, so come and watch because I'm about to prove you wrong."

She said, "Oh yeah, whatever."

And I said "Seriously, I'm about to show you something and if you don't think it's amazing, you will never have to work on me again because I've done this by myself so watch this."

She had this massive attitude with me and I didn't think she was going to get up and come watch me, but she got up with her sandwich in her hand and she walked over to the parallel bars. I did exactly what I just did moments before—I grabbed my legs out of the wheelchair, placed my feet down on the floor, did my preload action and I stood!

I looked at her and all she said was, "Oh, you're a bit taller than I thought you would be."

That's all she had. Only two hours before, she couldn't even hold me up. Between the three of them, they couldn't hold me up, but then I just stood up on my own two feet with my own energy, my own body, with no other help, and that's all she had to say to me.

I looked at her and I said, "Well your attitude still sucks, and I know you'll never ever look after me."

And that was it.

She turned around and said, "Okay," and started eating her sandwich again and walked off.

I called out, "This is fucked! This is seriously fucked 'cause you guys are meant to help. Why did you become a physio if you're not going to be positive?"

I don't know if she heard me or not and I didn't care because I was done with all of them. I had stood on my own and dragged myself the length of the parallel bars and back to the chair. I did it. And I did it all by myself.

I got back into my chair and went back to my room. I rang mum straight away and as soon as I heard mum answer and say "Hello," I started crying on the phone to her. I told her what I managed to do and what the physiotherapist said to me.

I said, "Mum, mum, guess what? I just stood! I stood in the bars by myself! I'm standing!"

My voice broke from tears of joy.

Mum was so excited and I heard her happy tears and the excitement in her voice when she said, "We did it! We bloody did it!"

Mum was so happy and so proud of me. I rang all my mates to tell them the new progress I made. It was the most exciting moment of my life because I was getting my life back and I knew it would motivate everyone to believe that the prognosis wasn't my life, and it was just words.

When Dingo and his mum came in to see me later that week, I saw them about to come into my room.

I said, "Stop, stop, wait."

They stopped at the door and asked what was wrong. I threw my legs out of the chair, grabbed onto the fridge, and stood up.

I said, "Check this out! Now give me a hug."

Dingo came over to me and gave me a hug. I saw the tears of joy in his eyes, and his mum was crying happy tears.

I said, "I told you I wasn't going to let you down."

He didn't know at the time that I could stand because I hadn't told him. I wanted to surprise him. I had come a long way from the day of the accident when he and Daniel witnessed me crash and break my neck.

All my family and friends were told that I was never going to walk again, and within two months I was standing. That's how I did stuff because I never wanted my friends to think they should worry about me. I thought that they blamed themselves in some way for what happened to me but it wasn't their fault. It was completely out of their hands. Dingo was about to head off to America and I wanted his last memory to be of me standing and giving him a hug instead of me being stuck in a wheelchair. And I was able to give him that.

# Kay

I was always excited when Josh achieved anything because his prognosis was "no recovery." So any progress, no matter how small, was fantastic. I gave him my words of encouragement and I was very excited for him. I could hardly wait to get over to the rehab centre to celebrate with him. I always knew he would improve even if it were just a little bit each day. Josh began to understand his body on a very intricate level. His knowledge assisted him with understanding what movement had to be done to achieve an outcome. Still, I was frustrated with the total lack of support from the rehab staff. That's why we started to bring Josh home most weekends.

It was time to have BBQs and friends over, and they arrived in droves and spent all weekend with him hanging out at our home just doing the things they normally did on weekends. It also provided the perfect situation for another member of our recovery A-team, Bing, to work her magic on Josh. Bing was trained in acupuncture at the Beijing Spinal Injury Hospital in China. Paula found her and believed she would be a huge help to Josh's recovery. Bing worked on Josh for one or two hours at a time on weekends at our home.

The weekends were all about Josh seeing life go on as usual and that he could get it all back. It was going to take a lot of work, but Josh was up for it.

My day of standing provided the sort of motivation that kept me going. I had a goal to walk and I managed to stand. There was no doubt in my mind that I was definitely going to walk.

It was coming up to my birthday and I thought, *I can't be in this rehab unit, I just can't. I'm not spending my nineteenth birthday here.*

So then I went through the laundry list of stuff I had to do to get out of there. To discharge myself early, I not only had to prove to the rehab staff that I could manage back home independently, but I also had to jump through all the paperwork stuff.

After eight weeks, my left leg started coming back to a point where I was almost strong enough to push myself around in the wheel chair with my foot on the ground. There was one boy in rehab with me who was a year or two younger, and he had a very similar injury to me. He also gained a lot of movement back even to the point that he could use crutches to get around. I hung around with him quite a bit and we fed off each other's progress, which helped the time in there go quicker. We messed around in the chairs a bit and caused a bit of a ruckus. We always tried to push the envelope and have some fun.

In rehab they had a hydro pool, which I couldn't wait to use. My first time in the pool, I thought I would be fine but I sank to the bottom like a lead weight, but once I gained my confidence, I loved it. Being weightless gave me the opportunity to try to use my legs and that gave me a lot of quick progress. It was just a pity that they only allowed us to use it once a week just for an hour, but in that hour I made sure that I used it to its full potential, whether it was floating with the physiotherapist moving me side to side to relax my body or doing small water aerobics. Just having the ability to learn how to stand in the water by holding onto the rails was amazing.

To discharge myself from rehab, I had to show the ability to self-manage my life. I had already moved into my own room at rehab and was pretty much self-managing three months earlier than they set the target for me to achieve, so there wasn't a whole lot I still needed to do. I just knew the sooner I got home, the sooner I would feel more normal.

I also redid my car driver's license while I was in rehab. Originally, the authorities wanted me to have hand controls but I wasn't having that. I went for the option where I had left foot controls with a device fitted to the car so that I could swap the accelerator from the right side of the brake to the left side of the brake. Leading up to the test, my mum organized to get my car brought into the rehab car park and left it there. When someone visited me, I went out and practiced my transfers in and out of my car. Having my car there was bittersweet. It reminded me of my old life as I sat in my car and smelled it, and saw my old CDs for the first time in months. It was so surreal and at first it made me sad, but once I started to understand how to transfer into it and actually sit in it, I got more excited and it gave me even more encouragement to move forward and never look back. Keeping my focus looking forward was the only way I was ever going to get my life back.

So that was it. I completed the last laundry list of tasks.

I arranged with mum for her to come and get me, and I discharged myself on 11 November, which was two days before my nineteenth birthday. Mum arrived in the early afternoon and I couldn't wait to get the hell out of there. I think mum couldn't wait either. We packed up my room and got all my things together. I pushed my wheelchair up to the sliding doors that I said I would walk out of when I first arrived at that rehab centre. I had a pair of crutches with me because I was still wobbly on my feet, so I had them to use for stability and balance. I grabbed the crutches and I stood up out of the wheelchair, and I walked out through the sliding doors of rehab with no hesitation.

Of course there had to be some twist—it couldn't be as easy as that! Just as I walked through the doors, my jeans fell down to the ground. I lost so much weight that my pants just fell straight to the floor.

I looked at mum and said, "I think I'll get back in the wheelchair now."

But I did it. It was probably the ugliest walk, and it was definitely the shortest walk, but it was the most important and meaningful walk I have done in my entire life. I was vertical on my own two feet and I walked out of there. I walked through the doors on my own two legs by using a pair of crutches straight out the doors I said I would walk out of.

Four and a half months later—July, August, September, October, November—just under five months to the day that I was told I would never walk again by all the doctors, physiotherapists, occupational therapists, and every other specialist, and there I was walking. I walked because I knew I would. Mum knew I would and I showed everyone that I would. I never gave up!

# Kay

When I think about the time Josh spent in hospital and rehab, I think how naïve we were and that ignorance was bliss. We knew so little about spinal cord injury but I just believed Josh would walk and he did!

Josh had a practical approach to achieving goals. Sometimes it was the smallest things he would figure out and it would work and triggered other actions and ideas.

I was so excited seeing him walk—it was amazing, I was so proud of him and naturally I took pictures! Of course the other great part was that we were over and done with rehab and Josh could continue his recovery in a far more encouraging and supportive environment with me, his family, his friends, and his very capable recovery A-team!

# Chapter 4

# If Strength is Born from Heartbreak, then Mountains I Could Move

## A loss is only a loss if you don't learn something worthwhile and better your life from it.

It had been several years since the accident—almost 10 actually—and life was moving along at a good pace. I was doing much better physically, mentally, and emotionally.

I saw my chiropractor Simon regularly, at least once a week, so he could continue helping me with my ongoing recovery. Even though almost a decade had passed since Simon first started my recovery program at the beginning of my accident, it was necessary to have him continue working on me to maintain my mobility, flexibility, and most importantly, keep my muscles stimulated and active.

On my latest visit, we talked about the incredible results I had achieved and how far I had come in my recovery from those early sketchy days in hospital when I was completely paralyzed.

The greatest achievement in my recovery for me was that I left the rehab centre upright, walking, and very motivated. Once I got home, I wanted to continue doing all the things I was doing in my life before my accident. I wanted to live my life as normally as I could. I wanted to keep improving enough so I could get back to doing all the things I loved to do before my accident. I wanted to get back to the mountain, get out onto the snow, ride down a run, feel the wind in my face, and hear the snow crackling under my snowboard. I wanted to get back on my motorbike, go for long rides, and go to motor cross events with my mates, but the reality of the last four or five months of everything since my accident that I had gone through and that my body gone through crept up on me.

I knew I had to stay focused and not lose sight of my goals and aspirations, so I got back into a regular gym routine. I decided not to adjust it to suit my injury though, because I had to keep my life as normal as possible if I was going to convince my mind that my life was continuing as normal as I was doing things that I would have been doing if my accident hadn't happened.

I always had to keep looking forward. I could never give up on new techniques, healing therapies, or ideas that gave any new improvement. Every time I got something new back, whether it was new sensations or movement, it always gave me such excitement and the belief that I would be okay no matter what.

As Simon and I talked about how far I had come in my recovery, over these past 10 years I realized the days, months, and years quickly disappeared. After years and of doing recovery work, watching my diet, keeping myself motivates and focused, I started to want to do more in my life than just train and visit Simon regularly for adjustments.

I felt like it was time to put everything that I had achieved in my recovery to the test—all the healing, all the training, all the adjusting, and all the movement that I had worked so hard to get back—and start to enjoy things in my life. It was time to be around my mates more, go out, have fun, and experience all the normal things that people in their 20s do, so that's what I did! I didn't want to have regrets by feeling like I was missing out on anything.

I started spending quality time catching up with my friends. There were so many in our group, but I could always count on Zayne, Laslo, Boz, Alex, and Ross being there for me. I had the best mates in my life and I certainly didn't have any problems letting loose and partying with the boys.

Our group's favourite haunts were Kittens and Bar 20. We nicknamed these clubs "The Office" and "Home" due to the long hours we put into both these places. We definitely knew how to party well into the early morning hours. I eventually lost count of the number of sunrises that greeted us when we walked out the doors from those clubs.

When I wasn't out partying, most of my time was taken up with the motor cross scene. There were tours and events that we all attended, and we even did a bit of travelling around the country with Motocross. Life was good and we were having fun!

Then one morning, I got a phone call that changed everything.

It was 5 April 2009, which was a Sunday. I had just come off from the usual Saturday-night-out gig of partying with my mates. I got home late, so my friend Zayne decided to spend the night at my house instead of going home to his place.

Getting a good night's sleep was something I never experienced again after my accident. But I wasn't one to sleep the whole morning away, so I got up around 8:20 a.m. and decided to go out for breakfast. I woke Zayne up, and he, mum, and I went to the café around the corner from our apartment.

It was probably just before 10 a.m. when we finished eating. Just as we were getting up out of our seats to head off home, my phone rang. It was my mate Lukey Luke. He was a stunt rider and he was down in Tasmania at the Super Bikes event with one of my closest mates, Judd, who was racing there. Judd was one of my team riders for the clothing company I had created called Black Money. He and Lukey were doing the circuits down there.

I thought it was a weird time for Lukey to call me on a Sunday morning. Usually, he would be out riding on the track by then, but I picked up the phone and answered the call anyway.

Lukey was crying! I could barely even hear what he was saying.

When anyone gets a phone call like that, everything around them slows down. I got that tight feeling in my chest and my heart skipped a beat. Unless it had something to do with Judd, I just knew there was no other reason for Lukey to call me and be crying like he was.

He said to me, "Woody, I wanted you to be the first to know. I didn't want you to find out on the Internet or any other way. Judd has just been in a severe motorbike accident and he's been killed."

This deafening silence came over me and I went completely numb. I looked at Zayne and I think he knew straight away that something was definitely not right. He had this concerned look on his face. He kept staring at me and waiting for me to say something, but the words just wouldn't come out of my mouth. I must have looked so emotionless because I was in that much shock. All I could do was stand there frozen in complete silence while I looked at Zayne and mum.

I finally said to Lukey on the phone, "Are you sure? Are you sure about this?"

And he said, "Mate, I'm sorry."

He just sounded so broken on the other end of the phone.

I looked at Zayne and managed to utter the words, "Judd's been killed."

Zayne and Mum both stood there and stared straight at me. I wasn't showing any emotion on the outside, but inside was a very different story. I actually thought I was going to keel over from the shock. I was still processing the words from Lukey that had come over the phone. I felt like I was in this insulated bubble and that everything around me was detached and still with no movement—just a deafening silence! It sounds weird to describe it that way, but it was like I was momentarily in another time zone. Time just stopped, and everyone and everything stopped with it for those few seconds when I heard the words that my best mate had been killed.

The silence was broken when mum asked me what I wanted to do. I couldn't get my thoughts together and I just wanted to get out of that space.

I said, "I want to go home."

I walked out of the café. I walked straight across the road to where I had parked my car—a utility ("Ute") small pick-up truck—on the opposite side of the street.

I didn't even look at what traffic was coming along the road. I wasn't thinking straight. Zayne ran across the street and waved at the cars, stopping them from knocking me over.

We had all come to the café in separate vehicles because my Ute was like one of those typical pick-up trucks with only two fronts seats in the cabin and the long flat tray at the back. Zayne offered to drive with me in the passenger seat. He could clearly see that I was in no state to be behind the wheel. I had barely made it walking across the road without being collected by oncoming traffic.

We only had to drive a few hundred meters to reach home. I told Zayne

I was fine to drive, so I ended up driving while Zayne was in the passenger seat. We travelled the distance home in absolute silence—I didn't talk to him and he didn't talk to me—we didn't know what the hell to say to each other.

When we got back to mum's house, I went straight in and called another one our friends. I can't even remember whom it was I called, but as soon as I spoke to them and I said the words out loud—"Judd has been killed"—I fell apart and my whole world turned upside down.

Judd and I had arranged to catch up with each other two days prior on the Friday when he was in Melbourne, but we missed seeing each other by about half an hour.

I spoke to him on the Saturday and he said, "Sorry mate, I missed catching up with you yesterday, but we can still catch up on Sunday or Monday."

I was excited because we were going to have lunch together. We would get to sit down for a bit, have a beer, have a chat, and just be in each other's company. We hadn't seen each other for a few months; even though we talked on the phone once or twice a week, it was so much better to catch up in person. Then to know that I would never get to do any of that with him ever again just broke my heart. Before him, I never had a friend die from a pure accident. I couldn't come to grips with the sudden loss of him nor the feeling that he was there only two days ago but now he was gone!

A week later, Lukey and I travelled to Maitland, which is just north of Newcastle in NSW, to attend Judd's funeral. His memorial service was a week after that in Queensland on the Sunshine Coast.

It all made me feel empty inside. At the end of the funeral service when everyone was standing around the burial site, his family and friends walked up to the grave and threw in some roses. As nice as the roses were, I wanted to throw in something different. It had to have meaning.

It had to say, "Yeah, this represents Judd and me."

I had a Black Money symbol necklace with me. It was a silver necklace that I designed and had custom made. Judd always wanted it and one time I told him that when he made me enough money, I could put diamonds in it and I would give it to him. I couldn't think of anything more perfect to leave with him than this necklace that meant so much to the both of us. I had never let anyone else wear it; the necklace was very precious to me.

I walked past his family over to his burial spot. I don't think his mum and dad noticed I was there at the funeral service until they saw me standing in front of them at Judd's grave.

Lukey held me while I stood there, which was just as well because I was crying so much that I nearly dropped and fell into the open grave.

I placed the necklace onto Judd's casket, and I said, "I'm sorry that I'm giving it to you like this, mate."

I spent a lot of quality time with his family. We talked together for ages about Judd. I had become really close with them, so it helped me to keep Judd alive in my mind by being around his family and hearing all the stories about him. There were plenty of those to be told.

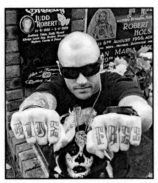

Some time later that week when we were all having lunch together, I mentioned to his family that I was going to do everything I could to make sure Judd's legacy lived on. He loved my clothing company Black Money as much as I did, so I thought about getting a memorial t-shirt designed to commemorate Judd. It would be a great way to represent something that was very special to us both. By having the Judd t-shirt as part of the clothing line, he would always be part of the brand as it carried on into the future.

Judd and I had so many plans about what we were going to do with my clothing line and how successful it was going to be. Even though it didn't feel the same without Judd being right there alongside me to share the excitement of watching it grow and expand, I wanted to continue with it and make sure I held up my promise to Judd's family—that his legacy would live on.

I didn't have any set plans, though. I really didn't know what I was going to do. I didn't have any money at the time and Black Money wasn't generating much income. The Black Money clothing range always sold really well, but it was small because I never had much money to support it. It was always tough to find money to keep buying more samples and to have designs done. At the time, it was pretty tough to keep it going with little money in the bank. While I was still committed to Black Money, I needed more funding, so I tried to figure out how to keep the brand running for a little longer to see if I could get the company back up on its feet and into profit.

Nearly to the day two months later, it was a Thursday morning when I was still in bed and my phone rang. It was a friend of mine, Bentley.

I thought, *Why is Bentley calling me this early in the morning? He must be on a bender or he has flown into Melbourne randomly and wants to catch up.*

I answered it on the last ring before it could go through to my voicemail. Bentley sounded terrible. He was just beside himself.

He said to me, "Woody, it's Bronte."

And I said, "What do you mean, it's Bronte? It's you, Bentley."

He replied, "No, no, it's Bronte. They think he passed away in his sleep. They're trying to revive him, but we're not sure if they're going to get him back."

"What do you mean?" I asked.

For a moment, I thought maybe Bronte had been in a car accident because he loved driving so much. That was one thing that gave him his freedom—being able to drive again.

Bentley said to me, "No, we don't know what has happened. You need to get down there to see Bronte. He's in Frankston Hospital."

I hung up and immediately rang Laslo.

I said, "You and I need to go down and see Bronte because they think he's going to die."

Laslo was at my front door within 15 minutes, which wasn't bad since he lived a fair distance away from my house. As soon as he arrived, we wasted no time jumping straight into my Ute and took off to the hospital. Mum and the girlfriend I had at the time went together in mum's car.

We took the freeway because at that time of morning there wouldn't be much traffic and we could speed along a bit. Mum was doing 100 kilometres an hour trailing behind me.

I just said to Laslo, "Fuck this," and I booted the accelerator and we sped off, leaving mum way behind.

I just wanted to get to Bronte. I thought that if this was going to be the last time I saw him, I just wanted to tell him that I loved him.

Bronte and I were very close. The first time I met him was at an after-party after a mini Super Cross event in Frankston. When the party finished, we went to my friend Brady's house. Bronte and I had a few beers and hung out there until 6 a.m. and our friendship just grew from there. The irony was that we had met just two weeks before Bronte had his accident.

He came off his bike while he was training at his home Super Cross track and he ended up with a spinal cord injury. Experiencing the same injury is what bonded us even deeper as mates.

In all these years I never had a mentor. I had never met anyone who had been on a similar journey to me, so we became very close. We knew each other; we really knew each other—what we were feeling, thinking, and seeing. I never had a connection with anyone like that before. I spent a lot of time mentoring other spinal cord injury patients, but I never let myself get close enough to anyone.

No one understood the pain I was in, no one understood the frustration I had, and no one understood the time or effort it took for me to do even the simplest of tasks on a daily basis. But Bronte did. In all the years I had to deal with my injury, this was the first time I could really speak to someone who just understood it!

Bronte and I couldn't just jump out of bed, throw on some clothes, grab a coffee and car keys, and be out the door in five. For us, getting out of bed alone took triple the amount of energy and time. People saw it physically on the outside but not the challenges and frustration we went through internally. Unless someone experiences having a spinal cord injury first hand, then they cannot possibly understand it. Bronte understood because he was right there experiencing it himself in exactly the same way as me.

There's that saying, "Walk a mile in my shoes," but I say, "Spend a day in my body."

It's what I feel—or more to the point, what I don't feel—not what others can see.

I remember when I first heard Bronte had his bike accident and was in the hospital. My mate Burnsey rang me and told me that Bronte was in the same spinal care hospital that I was in before. Bronte followed on in his treatment to the same rehab centre I went to as well.

I said to the boys at the time, "Well, I won't see Bronte until he's ready to see me."

They might have thought I sounded harsh saying that, but what people don't realize with me is that I don't go to see someone that has been injured unless they want me there. When I mentor people with spinal cord injuries, I explain to them that in order to gain the sort of recovery I had, it's a pretty tough road. I say some things to people that they don't want to hear or are not ready to hear, especially about recovery expectations, and the work required to achieve it.

Even though I was able to recover movement and walk in a certain amount of time, that doesn't mean that someone else is going to recover or walk in the same amount of time. I wanted to make sure that Bronte wanted me there, that he wanted to hear what I had to say, and was ready to hear it, because I can be the bittersweet deliverer of reality for some people. I waited until Bronte went to rehab before I made an appearance.

It was about four or five weeks after his accident, which was when we really clicked. We just spent so much time with each other from then on. We were both so committed with our recoveries that we did a vegan diet together where we only ate sticks and twigs for about forty days and forty nights. I called the food sticks and twigs because that's what it looked like. My mum and Bronte's mum sourced all this special food. It was completely vegan, which was funny because Bronte and I were big meat eaters.

Basically, the diet was a special blend of raw pulse foods rolled into small balls, which looked like rum balls. It was like super-charged organic wholefood. Apparently it helped regenerate the nerves and stimulated the whole nervous system and things like that. It was developed from an ancient recipe that was like a superfood. I struggled with eating it, but because Bronte was doing it, he kept me going. Once he had his mind set on something, he just did it, and I didn't want to let him down.

It was funny because I was supposed to be the one helping Bronte, but he ended up helping me more than anyone else—even more than I was helping him!

So Bronte and I only ate these little balls for forty days and forty nights. We didn't eat anything else, and the only fluid we could have was water. The diet was very tough on us both, but we were determined to see it through. By the time we finished the diet, we both felt better about our health. Our bodies were cleansed on the inside, but we decided that as much as we wanted to keep improving our health, we missed eating meat.

## Kay

A friend of mine told me about an American healer who was coming to Melbourne. We were always looking for different things to try because Josh was relentless in his search for answers that would help him gain more recovery. We had hit another roadblock and Josh was really just treading water. He was spending a lot of time with Bronte and helping him.

We went along to the American healer's presentation. The guy was dressed as a cowboy with a big cowboy hat. He was a real showman. We were sitting close to the front and we had a good view of him. He spoke about his mission with healing foods and something he said just clicked with Josh.

During intermission, Josh said to me, "Mum, I have to speak to this man. He can help me."

Josh wanted me to ask him a question but I said he had to do it. During the intermission, Josh and I spoke to him and Josh spoke very quickly about his situation. The healer was fascinated. When he came back on stage, he introduced Josh to the audience, and Josh told his story.

After the show was over, we spoke at length with the healer and his partner about the superfood he was promoting. Basically, he said that back in the old testament of The Bible, when the ancients went into the wilderness for forty days and forty nights, a group ate what was called pulse foods. This was food made up of certain plants, nuts, and fruits.

Until he came into the scene, nobody knew what the food consisted of. He had apparently studied the ancient scriptures and had developed this superfood. There were a few different versions. He sold them to everyone who attended that night.

His message to Josh was for him to eat the food for forty days and forty nights to see if it helped him. This was a huge commitment for Josh, but I have mentioned before, Josh was relentless in finding ways to gain more recovery.

Bronte and I always did things together. I introduced him to my chiropractor Simon, since he was a wealth of knowledge about the injury and how to manage pain relief. We always searched for better ways to manage our bodies through our injury. I even got Bronte to work with my healer Isabel and he got a lot out of her! It was cool how Bronte got into the healing that worked for me. All the boys got involved in helping Bronte as well.

We spent so much time together over the first year that I knew him. I shared everything I knew with him about our injury—what he could get back and how he could do it. After the first year, things started sinking in a bit more for him.

He stood! He could take really small rigid steps. He was always at it and he always tried new things. He had this carefree attitude.

He was like, "Well, I've been dealt this card, and I'm going to do everything I can."

He had this fight in him that I had never seen before, and it brought a greater fight into me. He never let anything get in his way from having a good time. He dressed like a "mad dog," and he acted like one too! He still did whatever he wanted to do. He didn't let his injury stop him but I knew it frustrated him because of the conversations we had. He always tried his best not to show it.

We both had our up and down days and sometimes we would say,

"We're fucking over it!"

And, "I'm just over this shit. I'm sick of being like this!"

When people heard that, straight away their knee-jerk reaction was that we were over everything. But we were just over it at the time. It was the frustration coming out, and in reality we knew it wasn't going to change and we just needed to fix it.

Bronte and I had these conversations about that all the time. Since we had the same injury, we totally understood what each other went through on a daily basis.

When Laslo and I arrived at the hospital, a couple more of our friends were already there along with Bronte's mum, dad, and younger brother. We were told that Bronte was on life support. I was gutted beyond belief. I just couldn't believe this was happening!

Not many of Bronte's friends had been told what had happened to him. Many of the boys were away on the Crusty Demons motorbike tour in a different state. They were halfway through a Harley ride from Mildura, Victoria, to Adelaide, South Australia. It would take several hours for them to get back and come to the hospital to say their good-byes to Bronte. Word of Bronte's condition spread quickly over the next few hours, and swarms of the boys started rolling in to the hospital. We spent probably 13 hours with him. Bronte's life support was turned off just before midnight. I was there with his family until the end—I was completely gutted.

Bronte was an organ donor and the doctors kept his body alive while the recovery team organized who would be the recipients, and his organs were donated to them. Even after he was gone, he still helped others. I was devastated and basically didn't come home for three days. I just chose to hang with the boys and grieve.

Bronte was from a small town in northwest Victoria called Kaniva. His funeral was so large that it had to be held in a big tent in the local football ground. Over 1,100 people attended. It was such a tough day for us all. Most of us had driven several hours to get there, so we all stayed in town for a few days and hung out together supporting his family and each other.

Both Bronte's and Judd's funerals had more than a thousand people attend. These two boys touched so many lives. I was already close with Bronte's mum, dad, and brother. I shared a special friendship with them because of the spinal cord injury connection.

After Bronte passed away, my world turned upside down. I had lost that other half of me. There would be no more bad sleep phone calls at 3 a.m. I always answered those calls from him because I knew how difficult it was to get a good night's sleep and I just wanted to help him in any way that I could.

After he was gone, I don't know how many times my body automatically woke up in those early morning hours from expecting a call from him. It was those little things that no one knew about our bond that left a huge void in my life.

I had to learn how to deal with Bronte being gone. I thought that if I distracted myself with something, it would keep me focused enough to keep away the pain of losing him.

I decided to re launch Black Money. I sold my motorbike. It was my pride and joy. I had just bought it and didn't even really get to enjoy it. I also sold a bunch of other things because I had to cash myself up.

A friend of mine helped me host a massive event—a "Night of Nights" for Black Money at his family's circus. We created a private circus night; it was so much fun. We had 300 people attend, and we followed it on with an after party. I had some special t-shirts designed and made in honour of the boys, Bronte and Judd. We framed two of them and auctioned them off, and the proceeds went to two of their charities.

Judd mentored a young boy who had health issues. We donated one of the framed t-shirts and $1,000 cash to this young boy. The framed Judd memorial t-shirt was bought by one of my best mates, Matty McMillan. He made the winning bid; he wanted the framed memorial t-shirt because he idolized Judd. Then another mate brought Bronte's t-shirt for $1,000 and we donated that money to Bronte's local motor cross club so that they could fix up the track.

That night, we also presented two other framed t-shirts that I had specially made to Bronte's and Judd's parents. Judd's mum and dad flew down from NSW. Bronte's mum and dad drove down to Melbourne from Kaniva, which is near the Adelaide border. I presented them with the new frames and t-shirts. I felt like I had done something to honour both the boys and add to their legacy.

And for a while there, everything started going really well again.

We had the successful launch in December with the Black Money brand of clothing and sales started to increase. Both the boys would have loved to see it take off again. They always had a lot of faith that the designs would really appeal and that the brand would take off. This time, I think I got just the right elements together. I had brought in two new designers, and the concepts they came up with were brilliant. They had really cool designs that took the overall look of the whole range to a new and fresh designer level.

Every year since I had started Black Money, we came up with a new look so it kept the line exciting.

Then, just when everything seemed to be going so well, an incorrect batch of stock came in that hadn't been cut to the specifications I requested, and everything changed.

This changed the whole shape and the overall look of the t-shirts. I was really upset about how they turned out. I had poured the last bit of my money into upgrading the website for the brand and to adding in more lines of apparel. We had created new designs for hats and bandanas, and introduced new brand items like stickers, sticker sheets, and graphic kits for motorbikes.

Even though our second year in the rerelease of Black Money wasn't as successful as the first year, we were still operating. It was a really hectic time. I was managing the company, and I had also just moved into a new house so I was busy getting all the furniture together for that.

All of this organization took up a lot of my time and energy, but it was great to finally be able to settle into my own space.

I just didn't have enough business experience back then. I did things like every time any of my mates came by, I let them have a few of each item—t-shirts, jackets, and jumpers—to take with them on their tours to wear so the brand was promoted. At first, it seemed like a great marketing idea to have Black Money clothing out there for people to see, but what I saw was more of my stock go down and no money come in.

Eventually, I didn't have the money to re stock, so I closed down the brand again.

I put all my focus back into setting up my house, and my Grandma helped me a lot with that. I spent so much of my growing-up years in her home that it only felt right that she was going to spend time helping me get my place in order. She was such a huge part of my life and she loved being involved in everything that was happening around me.

I loved her so much. I couldn't do anything without Dottie dearest being a part of it.

It was like reliving my childhood, only this time around we spent time together in my house instead of hers. We really enjoyed those moments of pottering around the place. Then she suddenly got really sick with cancer and I faced losing yet another special person in my life.

Dottie was like my best friend. She was an awesome lady—just a cool old school Aussie woman who spoke her mind and told us exactly what she thought of us. I just loved her. We all did.

She put up a brave fight with the cancer but she just couldn't beat it. She ended up passing away a day after the one-year anniversary of Bronte's death. This was another tough loss to cope with.

The only good thing with Grandma was that I got to say my goodbyes. I got to be there for her right up until the last moments of her life, so there was nothing left undone or unsaid. We got to say everything we wanted to say to each other.

## Kay

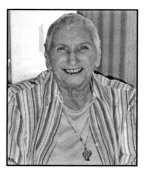

Josh loved my mother. She used to look after him a lot when I had to travel with my work. As he grew older he loved spending time with her. They would talk for hours. The older he got, the closer they became with one another.

When Josh had his accident, mum visited him all the time. It saddened Josh because he could see the sadness in her eyes. She never really got over his accident. When she came into the hospital to visit him, she massaged his hands and feet, and then she often just sat beside him and held his hand, and they would both sleep.

I had my sixtieth birthday in March 2010. It was a bittersweet day. All of our family gathered together to celebrate my birthday, but many there knew it would probably be the last time they saw mum.

Around the last week of May, the cancer really started to take hold of her. Josh saw Dottie as often as possible. She was admitted to hospital and then they sent her to the hospice. She was happy there. Her room was beautiful and overlooked the garden, so it was always filled with sunshine.

Josh often went to see her and spent quality time with her. I often arrived for a visit myself to find the pair of them asleep— mum in her bed and Josh sitting next to her holding her hand.

It was a Saturday morning. My cousins Mark, David, and Tim came to spend their last time with Dottie. She was really struggling to breathe and it was just devastating to watch her gasp for air with every breath she took.

In the end, we all told her that it was okay to let go and continue her journey, but she kept fighting to stay with us. That was so typical of Dottie. She lived for the family and she loved having us around her.

We stayed with her until about 10 p.m. Mum made me leave because I had a long drive and I had to get home to feed my dogs Montana and Thor.

I didn't want to go, but I had to. I knew it was the last time I would see Grandma. Mum and her brother left about an hour later.

Mum said to Grandma as she left, "Don't worry Dottie, I'll call you when I get home."

When mum got back to Port Melbourne, she called me and made sure I was home, then she rang my Aunty Wendy and Aunty Sue who had stayed at the hospice with Grandma. She told them that we were all home safely and to let Gran know.

Grandma passed away just after that call. I was devastated.

When mum and my aunts were going though all of Grandma's belongings days later, mum asked me what I wanted. I just said Grandma's floral recliners. I still have them; Montana and I love sitting in them. I feel close to Dottie when I sit in them.

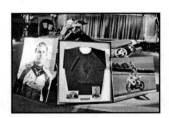

Grandma's funeral was held the following Friday. It was a dark rainy day, yet the funeral home was filled. We made sure that the day was about celebration, and we even managed some laughs. Dottie always loved a party. Later that night after the funeral, I went out to a local venue that I socialized at regularly. My mate Matty McMillan came with his dad Colin, who I met for the first time. Matty was the one who bought Judd's frame and the t-shirt at my launch and fundraiser that I had done months earlier. I had an awesome time that night with Matty and Colin, and we started spending a lot of time together from then on.

About four weeks later, Matty and I were at Kittens, our local Thursday night haunt. Usually if he was racing the next day, he didn't want to go partying the night before, and because this was also a weeknight, I don't know how I managed to convince him to come, but he did. I was surprised he was there partying with all the boys and spending his money. He was supposed to be putting all his money towards purchasing a new set of sport tires for his bike for the race.

We went to this same venue every Thursday night, although this time, we had a large group. There was about 16 of us. We had one of the best nights we'd ever had together. We let loose and had a ball. Matty was very sociable to say the least—he chatted up one of the girls at the club and took her home.

He called me the next morning and he told me, "I don't know where the hell I am, and I don't know what I've done, but all I know is I'm late for a race."

The next time I spoke to Matty on the phone, he was already down at Philip Island and was getting ready to go out on the track.

He said, "I'll give you a call Saturday as soon as I've finished the race."

He was awesome on the track. He rode really well. He got pole position just like Judd always did.

In those few moments just after he started his race, he missed slotting in second gear. He hit a false second and some of the other riders clipped him and he was knocked over and came off his bike. The group of riders travelling behind him hit him and he was killed instantly. I got a phone call from a guy that used to buy all my Black Money merchandise. I got to know him through the motorbike industry and because he bought my clothing.

I thought, *This is weird getting a phone call from the guy on a Saturday afternoon. I'll just take the phone call anyway.*

He said, "Woody I want you to know—"

And I thought, *Shit! I've got that phone call again. Oh no, there's only one dude that I know down at Phillip Island.*

And then he said, "Matty McMillan's been killed."

I said, "Matty who?"

I remember thinking, *Who is Matty McMillan?*

My brain wasn't allowing me to register the words I heard.

And he said it again, "Matty's been killed and we wanted you to know."

That was it for me! I lost it at him.

I said, "Don't fuck with me—no, this is not right! This is not fair! Don't fuck with me on this one!"

He replied, "No, I'm sorry mate."

The poor guy only wanted me to know what had happened before it hit the Internet. Facebook was so big and everything gets posted so quick. Everyone knew Matty was one of my best friends and they didn't want me to hear about it through the social networks.

When Matty died it crushed me. I was done now. I lost my three closest friends and my Grandmother all in that 18-month period of time. It was too much loss and too much grief to deal with. I was done with all of it. It just absolutely tore me apart.

After that, I just thought, *Everyone's just dying around me.*

My mate Peshy and I hit it hard after that. I think I did a three-week bender with him—a continual cycle of drinking, drugs, and strip clubs. It wasn't about using grieving for my friend's deaths as an excuse, but it was more about the fact that for the last 10 years I felt like I had always cared too much about what everyone else thought. I always had to be careful of what I did in case anything happened. I had to be careful when I partied—to not drink or do anything too much. I cared about what other people thought about me and I didn't want to upset anyone. The list of 'cares' went on and on, but I was over it!

When the boys went I remember thinking, *Fuck it! If I'm going to go, then I'm going to do what I want to do the way I want to do it!*

I didn't have any other means for an outlet. I couldn't snowboard and I didn't have a dirt bike, so in my eyes the only outlet I had was partying. That's why I hit it really hard. I hit it harder than able-bodied boys. I would walk out of the strip clubs at five, six, or even nine o'clock in the morning after having first arrived there about 13 hours before. I would go home, muck around with the dogs, have a feed, and then go back out and do it all over again. I did this continually for three weeks straight; I just went crazy. To this day, I still don't know how I didn't die during that time.

# Kay

For three years after his accident, Josh fought battles daily that would send a normal person insane, or at least into an abyss of depression!

Other than the morning after the operation, I have never seen Josh suicidal. Sometimes he was very sad, but I don't believe he was ever depressed.

For those first three years, which I believe were the crucial years that set him up for ongoing recovery, this 18-year-old man went from being full-on active to being trapped in a body and was only able to move his head and a little arm movement. All over again, Josh had to learn the very basics of movements that able-bodied people take for granted and don't even take a moment to think about.

Josh learned to sit up, rollover, and transfer from one object to another. He learned to stand and to commence using his hands. He fully committed to and embraced alternative healing methods—he learned how to meditate and do visualization techniques. He spent hours exercising his big toe through visualization and exhausted himself as he tried to get some movement back. Josh trained for four hours each week with a personal trainer at our gym, and for the other days he went to the gym on his own.

A friend once told me that years before she met Josh personally, she used to watch this young man wheel his chair into in the gym, get out of it, and relentlessly work out on weights.

She said, "He inspired me just by watching him."

She never forgot seeing him all those years ago as he worked out to get that bit better every week.

He gave up eating his favorite McDonald's meals and focused on nourishing food and no alcohol, even though he was a professional barman and loved alcohol. He drank cranberry juice until he hated it, and he learned to love nuts, berries, and even green vegetables. He ate pulse food, which was a special blend of lentils, grains, nuts, seeds, and dried fruits mixed together, for forty days and forty nights even though he was a carnivore. He only ate and drank all clean-living foods.

Then, when he realized that this way of being was a life sentence, he thought, Stuff it!

He did what he wanted and he partied. He even dabbled in drugs, which he took in social situations. While he took them to help him relieve his ever-present nerve pain, they also relieved the mental and emotional pain for him. He took them with great care in a controlled environment, such as in an apartment with friends there with him in case something went wrong.

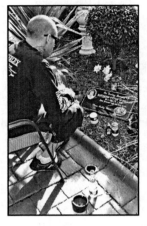 I wasn't happy that he had resorted to doing this on any level for any reason, but I was powerless to stop him at that time. All my threats to pack up and walk away from him and leave him to his own devices fell on deaf ears. It was a very stressful time for me to watch him. Thankfully, he soon realized that although the drugs helped the pain, it always came back.

So, he decided that there was going no easy solution, but he had to continue to find ways to improve and just learn to live with pain, which he described as, "All the time, never stopping, and like my body is on fire—it feels burned, and then on top of that he felt like someone is scraping their nails through my skin."

And this pain was 24/7—it never ended for him. He still feels it to this day.

So many people criticized him, and they also me because I didn't stop him from partying the way he did.

Although I wasn't happy, I understood it. There was so much Josh had lost in his life that he didn't get to experience anything that a normal young man gets to experience. During what should have been the best time of his life from when he was 18 into his 20s, Josh's life was filled with constant monitoring and restrictions every single day!

On top of all the grief he had to work through for his own life, he had the grief of losing those boys and his beloved Grandma Dottie.

The one thing that saved Josh was his ability to always refocus. He let himself go so far and then, just as quickly, he turned back around and pulled himself together to get back on his program.

I just used to say, "Well, he lost all those years that he was entitled to live, so what was the point of all his hard work if he didn't have some fun!"

My son is and will always be my wild child, but he is mentally tougher than anyone I know. He is inspiring to everyone who takes the time to get to know him. He is my benchmark for courage. Josh is my hero!

After everything he has been through and endured, he survived and he got through it all because he gets it! He understands, and he has more knowledge about recovery from this injury than anyone I have ever met. He never gives up!

Then a good friend stepped in and pulled me up. She could see that I was in a self-destructive mode because of my destructive behaviour. Peshy (Mark) was going over to China. He did stunt bike riding and he put on some shows and attended some bike events. He was one of my best mates. He was one of the ones I partied with so we always did stuff together.

When Peshy left, there was another void that opened up. He was the person I leant on the most, and he leant on me. With him leaving to go China, I felt like I was on my own and was dealing with everything all over again. I tried to fill the massive void by partying, and that's all I did—party, party, party!

The only thing that kept me from total self-destruction was my dogs and worrying about my dogs. Even then, I didn't take them to the park as much as I should have. I still took them two or three times a week, but I didn't spend as much time with them as I used to.

My good friend simply said to me, "Josh, you need to get away. You need to go see Peshy. You're not dealing with this properly, so I'm sending you to China."

She paid for my ticket and off I went to China to spend time with my mate, and get my head together.

Peshy did the Super Bike circuit and while there, I got to ride on the racetrack. I had never ridden on a racetrack before, but there I was, racing bikes on the racetrack with Peshy and Sammo.

I stayed for only a week, but it felt like a month. I wanted to catch up with Peshy to see how he was doing. I knew Matty's passing hit him very hard. They had a close friendship and Peshy was the sort of bloke that wore his heart on his sleeve just like I did. In fact, our birthdays are only days apart, so we share very similar traits.

He had a big smile on his face when I arrived at the airport. He had spent the night sleeping in the waiting lounge so that he could be sure he was there to greet me. He had been in China for about month by this point, and he was already making his presence known around the different circuits. He lived in Zhuhai, which is on the southern coast of the Guangdong province. It's a popular tourist destination and the surrounding area is beautiful. It has a completely different culture than other Asian cultures and cities I had been to before. I felt very comfortable there, and I thought it was the right place for me to clear my thoughts and refocus myself.

Sammo had been over there for about a year. He actually got Peshy the job of riding in all the circuits.

I got to ride the racetracks everyday. It was the best therapy I could have received. I recaptured all the excitement and freedom of being on a bike just like I used to feel before my accident. It was like my injury wasn't there and I could enjoy being on that track without any restriction.

I videotaped Peshy doing his stunt work. I had a scooter to get myself around so I wasn't dependent on anyone else. I loved that independence.

The city put on a fantastic nightlife. We partied like we did at home—we were out until all hours of the morning. It was great, and it was a relaxing environment. I felt at ease, so I was really able to unwind.

I was happy to come home because I was satisfied that Peshy was okay. Even though he missed the boys as much as I did, he seemed to be in good place mentally and emotionally. He had his stunt riding and he did well on the circuits, and he was happy.

I came home to the other boys, Zayne and Laslo, and it was coming up to summertime—our time to be at the river and go away for holidays. I knew everything was going to be all right—or so I thought.

Not long after I got back from China, there was more sad news. I saw it on Facebook actually. Another one of the boys from our bike-racing group had died. He had his accident the same time as Bronte's. In fact, he was in rehab with Bronte at the same time, so they went through their treatment together. This friend was in a wheelchair at first. Then just like

Bronte, he proved the doctors wrong and learned how to stand again with a frame. He had complications in his sleep, and unfortunately he passed away.

These two boys were really fit kids, and they always tried to get better. When this last friend of ours died, it was just shit. I had watched four families bury their kids, and no parent should ever have to bury their child.

It was a time for more reflections of those who had been so much a part of my recovery and now supported me in spirit!

I struggled to deal with all the loss and grief of the boys dying, and then my Grandma, and then this other friend.

I thought, *What the fuck's going on in this world? I've had all these people die around me.*

I didn't cope with all the loss. I knew I didn't cope with it, but I couldn't pull myself out of the spiral of despair. There was just this deep, deep sadness. I felt like my whole world had just crashed around me. Everything that had been the foundation of my recovery was gone; it was the most harrowing 18 months of my life.

Right up until the moment he passed away, I spent nearly every day with Bronte. We were like conjoined twins. Everywhere I went, he went. Everything I did, he did. When he passed away, it felt like a part of me went with him. This was someone who shared the most challenging experience of my life while he lived through the same challenge himself.

When I looked at Bronte, it was like looking in a mirror. We were so similar in so many ways. We also had our differences, but we shared the same injury, and no one understood what we went through every single day. I didn't have to explain anything to Bronte. He just got it! He knew it because he lived through it as well. He was just so inspiring to watch.

I felt that because I had the cord injury first, I was going to be the one who taught him how to cope with it, but he showed me. He just never let anything bother him, even if he had a toilet accident. That was enough to devastate me, but not Bronte.

I remember one night, Bronte, the boys, and I were all out on the town. There were about 20 of us and we ended up partying in the casino.

Bronte said to me, "Dude, I've pissed my pants."

So Burnsey and I took him outside in the wheelchair, and we put him in the back of my four-wheel drive. We helped him to clean up and change, and he tried to hit us in the face with the catheters and stuff because that's what he was like. Nothing fazed him.

When I went through an incident like that, I would implode. I would just become a mess.

I would shout and yell, but Bronte was just like, "Fuck it, whatever," and he didn't bitch about it.

That changed me as a person. It was inspiring to me; it sounds stupid to anyone else, but someone who goes through this injury understands that they have many moments where they feel like they can't control anything. But with Bronte, he didn't let his injury control him.

Instead, he would say, "Whatever, I'm not going to cry about it."

It made me think, *Man, this dude's awesome!*

I just loved him. I tried to cope with Bronte passing away only a couple months after losing Judd.

I was barely over the shock of Judd passing away, especially with the way he went. I had never lost anyone from a pure accident. It was just so quick, like when someone flicks a light switch—first he's there in full brightness and in living colour, then, *flick*—nothing but blackness. And I realized he was gone, and this huge void was created in my life.

Judd and I went beyond just being mates. He was very involved in my clothing business Black Money. He always wore the clothes to promote the brand and passed them around. He was one of my sponsored team riders, so he wore some piece of the Black Money clothing in every Super Cross tour he was on.

We shared the same passion of Super Cross and that whole motorbike scene. We would speak on the phone pretty much every second day. We had so much contact, and then it stopped—the phone calls, the catch-ups, having a beer, listening to our favorite music together—a huge part of my life stopped, and I never got to experience it again.

I wasn't prepared when my Grandma passed away either. She was like a mentor to me. I spent most of my growing years with her because mum worked long hours and travelled with work a lot. Dottie was just always there. I don't remember a time when she wasn't. I always knew where I stood with her because she always told me as it was. She was like that; she wasn't afraid to speak her mind. I think I inherited that same direct approach as well as her fighting spirit. Even though the cancer took hold of her, she never gave up fighting.

In 2009, on the night of my cousin Sally's engagement, my Grandma had to go to the emergency room at Frankston Hospital. She was coughing up blood. Grandma knew that the cancer she had beaten twice was back. She discharged herself from emergency and came to the engagement party. She always loved a party and she certainly wasn't going to miss a family engagement.

It was about two weeks later when it was confirmed that she had irreversible lung cancer, so her doctors started her on a palliative regime to give her more time.

Like mum and I, Grandma didn't hear the word *palliative*; she just heard treatment. She thought since she had done it twice in the past that she would beat it again.

Dottie taught me what real courage is. She taught me to never give up. I spent so much of my life with her—probably nearly equal to the amount of time I spent with mum.

She wasn't a typical grandmother. She was so cool, and she always supported and encouraged everything I did. I knew I could always count on her and she was there for me no matter what I needed.

There was a hotel near my Grandma's retirement village called the Tanti Hotel. As a special lunchtime menu, the hotel restaurant served oysters for half price, which made them more affordable. I drove from Caroline Springs where I was living and went all the way to Mornington where Grandma lived, picked her up, and took her to the Tanti Hotel for lunch. We had our oysters there and then I drove back to her unit. We sat on the recliners and chatted for the rest of the day, and then we often went to sleep. I loved those times.

I did the same when she was transferred to the hospice to see out the rest of her time. I just sat beside her and held her hand until she fell asleep. I often ended up falling asleep in the chair beside her.

The only good thing was that I got to say everything I needed and wanted to say to her.

I didn't have that same opportunity with the boys.

It didn't make the situation with my Grandma any easier to handle, but it gave me a different type of closure. This passing left a huge emptiness because it was with someone who was with me my whole life.

How do you fill emptiness that big? I was just devastated.

And then Matty went. It felt like I relived losing Judd all over again. Matty and Judd's lives were mirror images of each other. They were both passionate bikers, they were equally talented and successful in their events, and they both had larger-than-life personalities. They were such fun to be around.

Matty was just this very sociable fun-loving guy; he was the life of every party and he was really popular with the girls—they always chased him around trying to get his attention. Matty and I became very close, and even more so after Judd and Bronte were gone. Every aspect of our lives was spent together—socializing, following the bike circuits and events around the country, and training at the gym.

Matty's dad Colin often came to the gym and trained with us. The three of us went to clubs together and to the pub for a beer. Our whole social scene was spent together. We were like family.

When Matty bought Judd's framed t-shirt at the fundraiser event I held, it was like Judd was still with us and was living on through Matty.

Watching Matty at his racing events, getting pole position, and winning the races just like Judd did was like seeing a repeat of the same movie. So with both of them gone within such a short period of time and both in the same way, it freaked me out and really devastated me.

There was this invisible thread that kept me connected to all of them— through our passion and association for motorbikes, through our shared cord injuries, and through our family bloodlines. Then, this thread broke!

I was separated from all of them, and I felt a wave of sadness hit me. It took everything out of me—more than I realized at first. It felt like I was caught in a rip in the swell of strong seas and wave after wave came along and hit me harder than the one before it, and I was pulled under the water, and each time I struggled more and more to come to the surface. And even though I managed to, just when I thought I could catch my breath and get my bearings, BOOM! Another giant wave smacked me down again.

I wondered how many times could I get smacked down before I would say, "Fuck it, I'll just stay down."

So I just kept partying, because I didn't have to think about anything then. I was just on autopilot party mode.

Then around October or November in 2010, not long after my other friend had passed away, I was still partying all the time. After one particular night, I got home a bit late, so I slept in that morning and I woke up to find my two dogs Montana and Thor sitting on my bed beside me and they were staring straight at me. So I got up and went into the kitchen to get my breakfast ready, and they were both only one-step behind me. Then they followed me into the bathroom like they were my shadow. Then I went back to the kitchen again, and as I sat down to eat my breakfast there they both were, sitting as close as they could next to me, still staring right at me.

I suddenly realized why they were both behaving this way.

I thought, *I haven't hung out with my dogs for so long!*

I wondered if they missed spending time with me, and all the things we used to do together.

I used to go for drives with them. I would put Thor and Monny in my Ute to go driving and take them to parks. It was like just hanging out with my mates. I saw them as my children. They were my closest companions.

When I looked at them that morning, I could see the love and care in their eyes and I felt terrible that I hadn't been giving them the love and attention that I had given them before. I had the responsibility not only to care for myself, but also for two other beings, and that made me look at the way I was acting and behaving.

I started to pull my head in a bit after that. I started to clean myself up and I dropped the partying back to two nights per week and kept it respectable. I went back to the gym and carried on with my training, and I made sure I looked after myself and spent heaps of time with my dogs.

With all the backwards and forwards and letting loose, it just let me live without thinking about my spinal cord injury. I didn't have to think about training and I didn't have to think about what I ate because I just didn't care for four months or five months. I think it was something I needed to do and it taught me a lot, but I knew if I kept continuing down that path that I probably wouldn't be around much for longer to talk about it.

I remembered the boys and their families and my promise to keep their memories alive and keep their legacy living on, so I got back on track and became focused.

When Matty died, the boys and I listened to music all the time. I remember Peshy played me this song, and the song was called "Drones," which was performed by the band Rise Against.

One of the chorus lines is, "if strength is born from heartbreak, then mountains I could move."

That was when Peshy and I decided that chorus line was a tattoo that we both wanted to get.

I had my whole back and ribs done. The top part of my back is a big eagle and it has a human heart in its talons and it has smashed a skull. There's a giant skull positioned at the base of my back and it has been smashed in half. An eagle over a skull means "Victory over Death." That part is me dealing with my accident and moving forward. The heart represents my mates and my Grandma, and the love and strength I get from them. The eagle signifies honour and courage. It takes up my whole back.

On each side of my ribs, the writing says, "If strength is born from heartbreak, then mountains I could move."

With all the heartbreak I went through in those 18 months—losing four amazing friends and my Grandma who I just adored—with all that loss, I still managed to move forward and move all the mountains that could have stopped me.

## My favourite picture of Judd

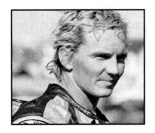

# Chapter 5

# We Found Love in a Hopeless Place

## Now we're standing side by side.

I got a phone call from my mate Maddo. He was up in Sydney doing a bike stunt at The Crusty Demons motorbike event.

He said, "If you're not doing anything, why don't you come up?"

I didn't really get to hang out with him very much when he was in Melbourne, so I spontaneously flew up to Sydney the next day.

Crusty events draw huge crowds and are really popular with both bike enthusiasts and the general public who want to see "Extreme Freestyle" motor cross. One of the big draw cards at every Crusty Demons show was the girls—the Crusty Babes. They are a group of models and dancers who perform dances and entertainment onstage at the shows at all of the Crusty events. I never bothered with the Crusty Babes because I thought they were all stuck up and that they had attitude. They wore tarty skimpy costumes but they were all pretty hot-looking girls with smokin' bodies.

Earlier that day in the afternoon, some of the boys and I went to Bondi Beach to hang out before the show. We met up with some of the Crusty Babes who performed in the show. Amelia was one of the Babes.

We were introduced, along with the other Babes, and Amelia and I talked for a bit and I thought, She's pretty all right for a Crusty Babe.

We all hung out for a while at the beach, then we headed back to the show, and I didn't think anything more of it. I stayed up in Sydney and partied with Maddo and the boys for the night, then flew home mid-afternoon the next day.

## From Amelia's Journal

### Introduction on the beach...

*Who would have thought when Josh and I initially met in October/ November 2010 on Bondi Beach (after being casually introduced by my friend), we would see each other again? Let alone get engaged 12 months later and then on February 16th 2013 be married!*

*Josh or "Woody"(as I knew him then), thought I was "just a Crusty Babe and they're all stuck up idiots!" How wrong he was!...*

*Yeah, he had an amazing story that I could relate to. Living with my brother who has autism and working with children with disabilities definitely helped me understand some of things Josh experienced on a daily basis ... Even though Josh doesn't have a mental disability, the attitudes, frustrations etc... are very similar!*

About two or three weeks later, Amelia messaged me. There was a book that came out that featured my story in it and she wanted to know more about my injury, what I had done in my recovery, and about me.

Her brother has autism. He lived at home with Amelia and her family. Amelia told me she was also a disability caregiver who cared for kids and young adults with disabilities such as brain injuries, Autism, Downs Syndrome, and Cerebral Palsy.

She was really intrigued about my recovery and she wanted to know more because she thought that the book might help some of the families to cope with children and young adults with these disabilities.

She started talking to me about it, and I thought, *This girl knows what she is talking about. She seems switched on and is very articulate and quite intelligent.*

## From Amelia's Journal

### Facebook did have a purpose!

*I guess I can thank Facebook too for bringing us together! If Josh and I never became "Facebook friends" after meeting on Bondi Beach, I would not have learnt about the book. His story was featured in The Well-Adjusted Soul and I'm glad I did find out about it, because*

I was able to purchase it, and pass it onto my Mum, and the parents of the children and young adults I cared for, to give them a little hope.

Amelia and I talked for a few weeks backwards and forwards on the Internet, and then I took a holiday break and went up to the river to Bundalong for the summer. I had been going up there for holidays and get-away weekends with my mates, Mitch and Shealesey, for years. They both had holiday homes up there and I always stayed with them. I was single and having fun.

I thought, *I'll bring the dogs up so they can have a holiday too.*

I didn't have any reason to come home; I didn't have to answer to anyone, so I went to my mate Shealesey's cabin and we just hung out for three weeks straight. We spent our time taking the boats out on the river, going into the town, having meals at the pub, and just lazing around the cabin.

## From Amelia's Journal

### November/December 2010

Josh and I continued to talk on and off throughout November and December and Josh learnt that I actually did have a brain and apparently I was an "ok chick, even articulate and quite intelligent"... Or so he said!

While I was up there, I talked to Amelia on the phone.

One day I said to her, "Well if you want to come up after New Year's, then come up and we can hang out and go on the boats."

So she came up, and we had the most amazing and fun two days together. I really enjoyed having her there with me. Then she had to go back home. When she left, I felt that because we were both single with no commitments, I didn't know if we were ever going to catch up again. I was just happy that we had got to share a few nice days together.

## From Amelia's Journal

### Into the New Year of 2011.

On 1/1/11 Josh convinced me to drive up to Bundalong (approx. 3-4hrs drive from home). We spent 2 days together, also with his friends and a friend of mine I had brought up with me. It was an awesome 2 days together but even then, neither of us knew if we would continue the friendship???

I personally, was on a path of destruction that was spiraling out of control!!!

Mentally and emotionally I was broken and not dealing with my own issues. I was out partying more nights than I was at home in bed and it wasn't unusual for me to leave home on a Friday night with a small bag, (big enough to fit clothes and make up in, but small enough to keep in a nightclub cloak room) and not return home until Sunday or even Monday!!! Sleeping at friend's houses in between partying.

I didn't think it was a problem... I was having fun and I didn't have to pay for anything because I was working for the nightclubs doing promos or dancing. I couldn't see that I was masking my issues with alcohol and the party life! I was totally happy on my own at that time, living my life without having anyone else to worry about. The last thing on my mind was having someone in my life.

Then a week and half later, I left Bundalong. Amelia called me as I was driving home. We had spoken a little bit on and off during that week.

I said, "I'm on my way home. I'll be home in a few hours—why don't you come over?"

She said that she was pretty tired from drinking, partying, and working all week, but that she might come over a bit later. She came over and spent Sunday night at my house, and then ended up spending Monday, Tuesday, and Wednesday. We hung out together from then on. We just clicked, and it felt like this massive void that I had in my life was filled.

# From Amelia's Journal

Back home from Bundalong...

Once I was home from Bundalong, Josh and I didn't really talk too much. I guess we were too scared to let someone into our lives. This continued for about a week and a half to two weeks until Josh then returned home from Bundalong.

The day he got home I drove from my Mum's house (in Melbourne's Eastern suburbs) to Josh's house in Caroline Springs (in Melbourne's Western suburbs) about a 1hr drive.

I was pretty tired from my reckless lifestyle, and I probably should have stayed in bed... (A very clear sign I was going nowhere fast!)

I wasn't the only one going this way... Josh too was on his own path of self-destruction after losing so many loved ones in a short period of time. I guess you could say we were a match made in destruction!

We had found someone that wanted to and could party as much as the other!

There were a few nights (to say the least!) filled with just that... In the city turning tables upside down, breaking glasses and blurring our minds of all that was hurting us deep inside. And we could, because we knew the club owners and security so we wouldn't be the ones to be kicked out!

We had no limits nor did we care. But from that day Josh came home from Bundalong, we never left each other's side.

Suddenly, I had this person in my life who took all the sadness away and filled the void that was with me for a long time. We just spent so much time together. There was something in me that knew after the first month that this was the girl I was going to spend the rest of my life with.

I was just excited about her, and about us, and about life. After that and without a second thought, I decided I wanted to marry her.

I was training with Colin McMillan (Matty's dad) at the gym. We had become very close and spent a lot of time together after Matty passed away. Colin became a father figure to me and I had an enormous amount of respect for him.

I said to Col, "Is it stupid if I propose to Amelia? We haven't even been together for a year yet."

I had this idea in my head that I had to be with a girl for two or three years before I really knew if she was the one.

I went on to say, "I just know. I just know that I'd be a dickhead if I let her slip through my hands."

Colin just looked at me and said, "Fucking oath, you should marry her."

And I said, "Alright, sweet!"

I couldn't wait to share the news with my mum. As soon as I got home from training, I rang her. She was in Ireland at the time, but I didn't care what the time difference was, because I just wanted to tell her my news!

I was so excited and I said, "Mum, I want to talk to you about something."

She said, "Oh what are you going to buy now?"

She had said that because that was the only time I would call her—to tell her I was purchasing something that I usually couldn't afford, but this time was different.

I said, "Well technically, I want to propose to Amelia."

## Kay

I met Amelia for the first time in Port Melbourne not long after Josh started seeing her. We had dinner in my apartment. Josh had many girlfriends over the years and several since his accident. Three of them had lived with us at various stages, so it was fair to say I didn't put myself out when I first met Amelia.

Our dinner wasn't as successful as any of us would have liked. Josh told me off for being a bit over the top about something we discussed.

Josh always used to say to me that I always criticized his girlfriends by saying they were never good enough.

I simply said, "When you meet a girl who looks at you the way you look at her, loves you for who you are, and accepts that you are injured and not disabled, then I will welcome her with open arms."

Amelia and her family came to Josh's talk on 16 March 2011, which was probably the first time I really noticed her love for

Josh. From then onwards, I knew they would be together forever. Amelia also became very close to our dogs Montana and Thor and they loved her.

I was travelling through Europe with my sisters and we had just arrived in Ireland.

Josh rang me and said, "I have something ask you. I want to propose to Amelia on my birthday and I want your blessing."

Josh's birthday was the day after I was going to return from the trip, and he had organized to have his party at a friend's bar in Prahran.

I suggested to Josh that he should see our friends Antonia and Robert who owned a jewelry business near Black Rock about the engagement ring. He did visit them. They were so excited to see him after all these years. They made a ring for him and we picked it up on the way home from the airport.

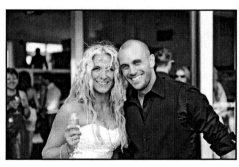

Mum went really quiet on the phone and I thought, Oh no, what is she going to say?

Then she started crying and she said, "That's fantastic! I know you are going to be happy with her. She treats you right and she always looks at you the way I wanted your girlfriends to look at you, and none of them ever did. But the way she looks at you, I know she's the right one."

As soon as mum said that, I thought, Sweet, I'm definitely doing it!

# Kay

From a mother's perspective, one of the biggest problems this injury causes is with relationships.

When Josh first had his accident, the room was always filled with beautiful young 17- and 18-year-olds that were there to support their injured friend.

In the first few years after Josh's release from hospital, he had a few girlfriends who were all committed but in those early hard months there was so much pressure and frankly I preferred him to be on his own rather than have the pressure of a relationship that was difficult at best.

He needed to focus on his recovery without complications, so it was very hard in those early years because Josh was very fragile health-wise. Fortunately he had some amazing chick friends so he was never without a group of gals around him. As he got stronger, he had some of what I guess he would have called longer-term relationships, but in my opinion, I could see that they were one sided.

I remember Josh saying to me, "You always criticize my girlfriends. They are never right in your eyes. Mum, you are so tough."

I would always say the same thing, "When I see them look at you the way you do with them then I'll be happy and be very supportive."

Over the years since Josh's accident, he had two or three long-term relationships. While I was always supportive, I felt that the girls weren't as committed as Josh was. Some were outright mentally and emotionally destructive.

I kept saying to Josh, "When the right girl comes along, then I will never be critical—I will be happy."

It is so hard to deal with this injury and all that comes with it, but when Josh met Amelia, it was apparent really quickly that they would be together forever.

Josh is a very traditional man. He is protective, loving, and will be an excellent father, and Milz (our nickname for Amelia) will be an excellent mother.

They are devoted to each other and I can truly say they are best friends. Josh's health issues in 2012 were so frightening, devastating, and confusing. I would not have blamed Amelia if she bailed out. Josh even said to her that she should go if she wanted to and that he would understand.

Amelia's love was so strong and I really believe it gave Josh the grit and determination to recover and be stronger than ever.

I am not saying it has been easy getting over the issues of March, April, and May in 2012, but with their love, and with finding more people including the amazing Uschi (in the USA) to bring into our healing circle, Josh emerged stronger and more focused than ever.

Josh and Amelia are both so happy, and although financially it has been very hard, they are getting through it and it's exciting to see them grow together.

For the first time in 13 years, I am really confident about the future because I know that Josh and Amelia are together and happy, and of course, that the doggies Montana and Thor are also happy and contented.

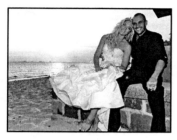

I wanted to keep it a secret and I didn't tell anyone—well, the secret lasted about an hour. I rang my stepbrother and my dad and then I rang my mates. Laslo was the first mate I called.

I said, "Las, I've got to catch up with you."

I thought that if Laslo thought it was a good decision, I would know I had made the right one even though I had already made up my mind to marry Amelia. I was just so excited about it that I wanted everyone else to be excited about it. So I met up with Laslo and told him my exciting news.

He said, "Fuck yeah! That's mad!"

I knew I was set then, and the next person to tell, or ask rather, was Amelia's dad. I arranged to have a Sunday lunch at the pub with Amelia's family. Originally I had the idea that I would just hang out at the pub with Amelia's dad Malcolm and have a few rounds of drinks together but it didn't work out that way!

To my surprise, the whole family was invited, so I just went with it.

When I first met Malcolm six months earlier, we met in the pub. At that first meeting, we drank about ten pints of Guinness each.

He had said to me then, "I'm glad my daughter has you for a partner, because now she has found someone who can drink as much as I can."

The funny thing is that back then on that first meeting, Malcolm and I talked about marriage and kids but I hadn't even talked about it with Amelia.

So on that Sunday, I sat in the pub with Malcolm, and then Amelia, her mum Jude, and sister Laura arrived. It was unusual for them to come to the pub especially on a Sunday afternoon.

I sat there thinking, *How the hell am I going to ask her dad for permission to marry Amelia with all the family here?*

I knew as soon as her mum and sister found out that they wouldn't be able to hold back. They would blurt something out to Amelia and my surprise proposal would be ruined.

Amelia and I had brought the dogs down in the car, so I asked her to take the dogs for a walk. I knew I had only a small window of time to ask Malcolm.

Just when I was about to ask, Amelia and Laura came back with the dogs, and in my panic voice, I said to her, "Take the dogs for a bit more of a walk."

She gave me this look as if to say, *What is wrong with you? I just took them for a walk.*

But thankfully, she did again.

I knew this was the moment!

I quickly said to Malcolm and Jude, "Jude, I didn't want to say this in front of you because I wanted you to be surprised. I want to ask for your permission to marry Amelia. I want her to be my wife. I want to marry Amelia! I know it's right, and I know it's quick, because we've only been together for 10 months, but I just know it's right. I love her so much and I will treat her right and I know she will treat me right. We will always have each other."

Jude started to cry.

Malcolm said to me, "Well, can you make babies?"

And I said, "Yeah of course I can!"

He replied, "Well then, you've got my permission because I want a happy daughter and lots of grandkids."

The girls came back from walking the dogs. Jude was crying while drinking a glass of champagne, which is really funny because she doesn't drink alcohol. I was worried that Amelia would ask what was wrong with her mum, and that Jude wouldn't be able to hold back and she would let the secret out.

When Amelia has come over, I said to her straight away, "Can you get me a beer please?"

And she said, "Is there anything else you'd like me to do?"

She didn't realize I was trying to keep her away. Laura sat down next to her mum. She was quick to notice that Jude was crying.

"Why is mum crying?" Laura asked me.

I quickly said, "I've asked permission to marry Amelia. I'm going to propose to her on my thirtieth birthday, so you better get your mum out of here before Amelia sees her and asks what's going on."

And then Laura started crying!

I thought, *I'm not going to able to keep it a surprise from Amelia.*

So finally, I managed to get both Jude and Laura out of the pub, so the secret was safe for the time being.

Over the next few weeks, I shared my news with family and close friends. Everyone was as excited as I was about me proposing to Amelia. I couldn't believe that we all managed to keep the proposal a secret from Amelia until the night of the "Today Tonight" interview. "Today Tonight" is a current affairs television program in Australia.

For several weeks they had been filming my recovery story and then they had heard about the proposal. It was a great way to finish that taped interview with Amelia, mum, about 75 of our closest friends and relatives, and with the camera crew and news reporters from the television show.

I discussed with the television reporters a couple of weeks prior to the taping about having a positive spin on my story. I told them I was going to propose to Amelia in two weeks. They extended doing my story so they could film me proposing to Amelia on my thirtieth birthday.

## From Amelia's Journal

### We are TV Stars!

November 2011 and "Today Tonight" decided to do a feature story on Josh! Yay! Finally, he was going to get the recognition he deserved and hopefully the right person would be watching that could help Josh continue his recovery. They did a few weeks of recording and then they decided to wait for Josh's Mum Kay to return from an overseas holiday she was on with her 2 sisters, Wendy and Susan (they were due home in 2 weeks time) so they could also capture her journey, as far as Josh's recovery was concerned.

They mentioned that they wanted to film Josh's 30th birthday celebrations at a local bar. As far as I knew, they just wanted to get some footage of Josh in a social situation with all of his friends... Little did I know the REAL reason everyone was being gathered there!

# From Amelia's Journal

### It's party time!

A few weeks rolled on and then it was Josh's 30th! Everyone was having a great time and I was enjoying catching up with family and friends we hadn't seen since coming home from America.

Then speeches started... I turned to listen to Josh talk like everyone else did... Except... Josh didn't want me listening in the crowd with everyone else... He insisted I went up and stood next to him!

Initially I thought "Why does he want me up there?" But I just shrugged my thought off and went and stood next to Josh as he insisted.

He started his speech with, "I'd Like to thank everyone for coming today" and then I noticed the "Today Tonight" camera crew come around the corner and before I could totally register what exactly was going on, there was a big furry microphone and camera crew in front of us!!!

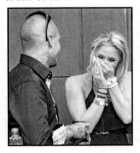

I looked at my mum and my friends and saw them all smiling and then I noticed they all had tears falling down their faces... THEN I heard Josh say, "Not only did I want you all here today 'coz it's my 30th, I also wanted to ask Amelia" and he turned to me with a ring in a box and asked, "Will you marry me?"... I was speechless!!! It must have been about ten seconds before I realized I hadn't responded and then I yelled "YES!" Then the celebrations really begun!

We celebrated that much that Josh and I didn't even see each other until it was time to go home.

One thing I had noticed, was Josh getting down on his knee a fair bit leading up to his 30th and I asked him, "What are you doing?" and he said, "Just stretching my hip flexor." I thought nothing of it because it wasn't unusual to find Josh on the floor trying to ease his pain with stretches... Now I know what he was really doing was practicing getting down on one knee to propose! Sneaky! Unfortunately he couldn't do it on the day because of where he was standing. If he bent down the camera crew would not have been able to see him because he would've been behind a large pot plant!.. But the intention was there.

Instead he came into my work the next day and recorded getting down on one knee and asking me again "will you marry me?" so he could post for everyone to see that he in fact could get down on one knee...!

## From Amelia's Journal

### The Big Wedding Day Arrives!

February 16th came and it was the big Wedding Day!!! The day I got to marry my best friend, soul mate and love!!! I had the perfect morning with my bridesmaids and it been a beautiful 38 degrees (Celsius) in Melbourne. Everything was just perfect! After all of the stresses I had planning this amazing day whilst in America I couldn't of possibly done anything better!

When I arrived I could see all of the Harleys lined up, Josh as expected turned up with the boys riding Harleys (Yep!, He still rides dirt bikes and Harley Davidsons all unmodified), as I stepped out of the car I could see Josh and the boys all lined up at the end of the isle with the beautiful Port Melbourne Beach behind them. It was time to walk down (we danced down) the aisle. I was so excited to get to the end I think Dad hit a slight jog!

And so the vows began:

"Most people wait a lifetime to meet their soul mate. Some meet as teenagers and grow old together still holding hands, yet others find their future partners in a variety of circumstances and these relationships stand the test of time, whilst others crumble or fail...

Amelia and Josh's relationship is based on mutual love, respect and a readiness to understand, accept and adjust to each other.

They don't accept the notion that one has to be subservient to the other, or that happiness can be achieved by one trying to change the other. These two have committed themselves and because of this, they may influence each other, and that can be a mutually enriching experience.

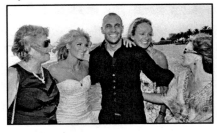

They acknowledge that marriage understands and forgives the mistakes life is unable to avoid. Equally they also acknowledge the vital importance in a successful marriage of willingness to compromise and share not only that which is good and enjoyable but also those aspects of life which are challenging and unpleasant. Above everything else that they are to each other, they are first and foremost each other's best friend, confidant and soul mate."

During the vows I noticed Josh needing water but I just assumed it was from the heat and the fact he was in a black suite and probably nervous.

It was the most amazing day EVER!!! It was a celebration of the love we have together and we got to do it with all of our closest friends, family and even our babies Monny and Thor (the dogs)!

Funnily enough, Josh and I hardly had a drink it was so busy and went so fast that we drove people home at the end of the night.

When we got back to the hotel, Josh told me that he didn't actually think he was going to make it to the wedding!!! Apparently after having a few drinks with the boys the night before (although he was very conscious to drink water also), he was dehydrated when he woke up that morning. As a result, he started to have the jolts! ... And quite a few of them I was later told!

So in a state of panic, the boys went to get electrolytes, food and water to snap him out of it. They didn't want to call Kay and worry her and they certainly didn't want to call me!!!

So Josh was trying to think of a way to get himself to hospital and out in time to make the wedding and not let anyone know. Very typical of Josh!

Luckily, when he collected the Harley from his stepbrother and rode it back to the hotel, the fresh air and concentration he needed to ride the bike snapped him out of the jolts. I know my Dad was relieved by this stage as he was worried about Josh's health.

...It's fair to say that Josh never gets a day off from his spinal cord injury and his injury doesn't care if you're getting married or having a day at home. It still controls Josh in many ways... I just hope he gets a day off when I'm in labour!!!

## Kay

The early afternoon summer weather was displaying its stunning best.

The beaches were full of sun worshippers. It was hot, the sky was clear, and there was a light breeze blowing off the bay, which provided a cooling effect for the afternoon's celebrations.

I text messaged Josh and Amelia that everything was perfect "beachside."

My sisters Susan and Wendy, Bali sister Asri, family friend Ray, cousin Richard, grand niece Ivy, and myself were all dressed in our fineries and travelled by maxi cab to the venue.

As we arrived at the restaurant, the Sandbar Beach Café, the staff were putting the finishing touches on the venue. It looked exactly like we wanted: casual, friendly, and beachy.

It seemed like everyone started to arrive at the same time. Then, we heard the Harleys rumbling down the road.

Josh was riding a Harley with his great mates Laslo, Wicksie, Paul (Dutchy), and Shaun riding their Harleys escorting Josh right into the venue.

The entrance was dramatic and the bikes took centre stage. There were cameras and smartphones taking pictures in every direction. The groom's team of Chrisso, Daniel, and Laslo looked fantastic all dressed in black. Everyone looked amazing and fresh considering the heat.

Josh walked over to me and said, "Thought I was off to hospital this morning. I thought I was having another seizure. Thank God the boys helped me out. They have been great today."

I asked him if he was okay. He said yes, but needed to really hydrate himself. I rushed inside the Sandbar and got bottled water for him and the boys to keep them cool and hydrated. I was between joy and panic. Josh said he was sorry that he had to tell me about the health scare he had in the morning.

He didn't want to tell Amelia and risk panicking her, so I got the news instead. I guess he needed to warn one of us in case something went wrong.

Pictures were taken, then the party moved inside waiting for the gals to arrive. The girls came in and it was a very casual walk down the makeshift aisle where we all gathered. Everyone looked so beautiful and the children were so cute. The bridesmaids looked amazing in their pastel colors.

Then Milz came in. She was a picture of beauty in her gorgeous gown. Her father Malcolm and her entered the marriage area. We all strained forward to listen to what was being said. The breeze had come up slightly but it was still blazing hot. The bridal party just looked stunning with the sun shining down on them.

It was hard for me to relax and enjoy the service since I knew about Josh's situation. I just watched him and frankly, I prayed for it to be over. I kept moving between the feelings of fear, joy, and happiness—it was hard to explain. I watched Josh's every movement, looking for a tell tale sign if anything was amiss. It was the most vulnerable time as Josh was standing in the sun dressed in black, which probably wasn't the best color choice to be standing in the hot blazing sun but he seemed happy.

There were a few times when he looked like he was struggling to focus, and at one stage when he was holding Amelia's hands, he asked for water. I prayed for everything to be okay and I tried to figure out what we would do if he had a seizure.

We finally got through the service and everything was fine. Yay! Relief! I could relax now.

The photographer asked Josh and Milz to stroll towards the pier so he could capture the stunning backdrop of scenery in the photo.

Josh just said, "Sorry mate, no can do. These aren't all terrain legs and it's going to be a huge day."

He was determined to not use his walking stick, which was long gone. I have watched him struggle to make his broken body work when it just won't play the game. This injury never discriminates.

Even on this special Saturday—during his wedding and walking in the sand—which is a surface that is very unkind to him to balance on, and he hates to walk on it.

It was around midnight when everything came to a close at the Sand Bar Café. Everyone said their final congratulations and goodnights to Josh and Amelia. I am sure that the three boys who passed away were standing behind Josh to make sure nothing went wrong. They always have his back. And my Mum, Dottie dearest, who I am sure was floating around. She was never one to miss a celebration!

All our friends and family came together as one with the same goal for it to be a memorable day for us all—and it was!

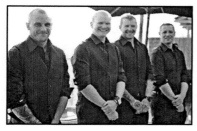

The Friday night before our wedding, Laslo, Chrisso, Dan, Patrick (who flew from Switzerland just for the wedding), and I were staying in a hotel for the night. We started having celebration drinks around 3 p.m. and didn't stop until about 11 p.m.

We didn't leave the hotel the entire night, and that's what I wanted—some time with my boys—to talk with them about anything and everything and just chill out for the first time in over a year. I could even have a drink and enjoy it without feeling sketchy.

The next day on my wedding day, I got up early to shower and do my morning duties. As soon as I stood, I didn't feel 100 percent. We had drank a few beers the night before and I didn't think much of it, but just to be sure the alcohol didn't affect me, I did also start to drink a lot of water straight away.

It wasn't until we went down to Chapel Street for breakfast when the fear kicked in. Just before we started to eat, I had a massive jolt—not as bad as the one nearly 12 months prior, but enough to put that same fear into me. The boys noticed it and they asked me straight away if I was okay, because they knew all too well what that meant.

I just brushed it off and said I needed to eat and drink more water. I'm pretty sure the boy's eyes didn't leave me the entire time.

I experienced a few more little jolts, and the time was getting shorter between each one. I didn't know what to do. I knew if I called Amelia to ask where the spray (a special spray to stop the Dysreflexia) was, then she would know exactly what was going on and it would ruin her big day.

There was no chance I was going to do that, so my next thought was, *How can I get to hospital without Amelia knowing?*

That was going to be too hard to do too.

As we walked to the car, Laslo offered to drive, but I knew I needed to get my mind off the worry and focus on something else, so I drove. We went to a few chemists but they didn't help, so Dan bought some strong electrolytes. We all needed them anyway. We went back to the hotel room and watched television and just chilled out. After two hours, I started to feel better. Then we had to go out to my stepbrother's place to pick up his Harley so that I could ride it to the wedding.

When Laslo and I rode back into the city, I guess the wind in my face and the fun of riding took away the fear of the jolts and I started feeling a lot better—not 100 percent, but the fear of needing to go to hospital had passed.

Once we got back to the hotel we all started getting ready. My good buddy Joshy Cachia turned up, then Zayne and Adam arrived. Shaun and Wicksie roared in on their Harleys, and lastly Dutchy arrived on his.

This was when the nerves started kicking in and the excitement of the wedding started to become very real. I was still a little worried about the jolts. I just didn't want any dramas through the ceremony. The last thing we all needed was our big day ruined by a hospital visit. I wasn't going to let that happen.

We jumped on the Harleys and took off to the venue and made sure everyone knew we were coming.

When we arrived, most of the guests were out at the front filming and taking pictures. As soon as I kicked the stand out for the bike, I was so relieved we all made it and made it there in one piece.

Not long after I got off the bike, Amelia arrived in Toddy's Chrysler 300, and the bridesmaids followed in Laslo's matte black 300C. The cars looked so awesome. We quickly went inside. I drank about two bottles of water and waited at the end of the aisle for the girls to walk in.

As Amelia got out of the car, the breeze flicked up her veil and it gently moved about in the wind. I could have burst out in happy tears right then and there, but I held it together.

She looked so amazing, and the girls looked great. They danced down the aisle to Rihanna's song "We Found Love." We chose that song because the lyrics suited our story of how we met and the self-destructive lives we were living two years prior.

Amelia was the most stunning bride I have ever seen.

She just glowed, and I remember thinking to myself, *How the hell did I pull such a smokin' hot wife?*

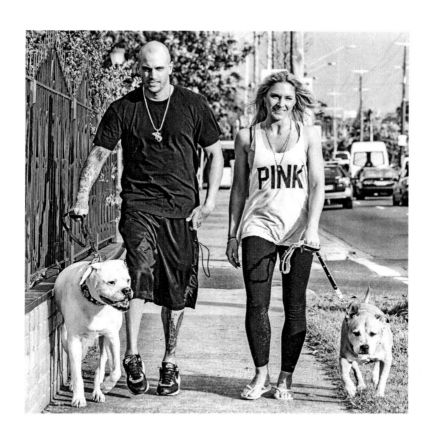

# Chapter 6

# Help Woody Ditch the Stick

## You go through life getting attached to different things, but it was time to ditch one of mine.

### From Amelia's Journal

Out of control!

I realized that I had been living a very 'out of control' lifestyle for well over a year. I had somehow managed to keep myself together enough to do my casual disability care hours and learn all my dance routines for the Crusty Tour (where I met Josh) but once I was on tour the party just continued!

I was partying and drinking too much and my eating habits were all over the place and I realized I needed to get them right to continue my life as a dancer... (Let's not forget I have been a dancer for most of my life... ever since I was 3.5 years of age).

So initially I was on the hunt for a nutritionist but got recommended to a personal trainer who also worked out your meal plans. It wasn't until my first meeting with them when I was asked, "How much alcohol do you drink?" That's when the reality of what I had been doing to my body hit!

New Training... New eating.. New program!

I started my new training and eating program and promised I would not drink alcohol! Yep... That's right... No more alcohol! This program was very successful for me... So much so that I went on

to win a bikini competition! This was the turning point for me!
Clean eating—Clean living! It obviously left an impression on Josh
because he started to clean his life up too! He was really committed
to clean eating and started to train on a daily basis. He also did
weight training with Colin McMillan at least four times a week!
This training was fantastic for Josh physically and mentally.

Josh mentioned that during his training sessions with Colin, they
would have their 'boy chats'... I thought it was great they were
building a father—son bond between them... It was something they
probably both needed. I'm sure this was guided by Matt (Colin's son
and Josh's best friend who passed from a horrific bike accident). It
was probably during this time of clean living that Josh and I both
realized, even though initially, we were totally happy living our 'out
of control' single lives, we held the same responsibility and were
accountable to keeping each other healthy and focused as we held
for our individual self.

We had actually been made soul mates whether we liked it or not!

I was really proud of Amelia. She completely turned her lifestyle habits
around and started eating really healthy and balanced meals. She went
cold turkey on drinking alcohol and picked up her training at the gym.
She got her body into such great shape that she won a bikini contest.
Amelia was smokin' hot and very healthy. She inspired me to get my act
together and I started a whole nutritional and training program of my
own.

Matty's dad Colin and I had grown really close. He was like a father
figure to me and he was helping me with my gym training and getting me
to be the healthiest and fittest I had ever been.

I had heard about a program called Project Walk in Carlsbad in
California. My chiropractor Simon got onto the website and he messaged
me to get on the site and check it out. I didn't take it any further at that
stage because I was a bit wary of rehab programs after my experience at
the rehab centre I went to after I was released from hospital.

A couple of weeks later, mum brought it up in a conversation, so I
thought I better give it a look. It was advertised as a state of the art facility that runs activity-based recovery programs for spinal cord injuries.

They also provided education, training, and research and development programs. When I watched the video and saw the results they received from working with spinal cord injured people, I wanted to jump on the plane right then and get over there. Only issue was the cost. I needed to work out how I was going to get enough money together to go.

## From Amelia's Journal

### Help Woody Ditch the Stick!

Josh was introduced to a program called Project Walk in Carlsbad, California by his chiro Simon. Initially, Josh wasn't interested because of his previous rehabilitation experiences, and honestly, who could blame him? Those experiences were horrible for him. As soon as Josh watched the video of how Project Walk worked he wanted to go. And of course Josh being Josh, he wanted to go yesterday! But of course these things don't come cheap, so "Help Woody Ditch The Stick" was born.

"Help Woody Ditch The Stick" was the name I came up with for the fundraiser to get Josh to America. I just knew Josh wouldn't ask any of his friends for help, so I did! I made the Facebook page and I invited everyone we knew! I asked all his friends to make donations of items that we could auction. They were only too happy to help Josh out. We ended up with a great range of items to auction off between the boys and Josh, from their signed motor cross gear to his tattoo artists artwork and tattoo hours, signed band jackets, car racer's gloves and cricket bats... And with the voluntary help from Josh's Mum, his Aunties and the Mothers of some of his friends and many more wonderful people, the night ended up being a huge success! We ended up raising about $18,000 (nearly the total amount needed) to go towards getting Josh to America for the recovery program.

Although I thought Amelia's idea to raise enough money for me to go to Project Walk was great, I didn't really feel comfortable putting on a fundraiser event where only I benefitted. I just felt that at the end of the day it was my accident, it was my fault, and it was my responsibility to pay for this opportunity.

I realized mum had been carrying me financially for so long and she was burnt out with money. So all the boys put money, donations, and items in to be auctioned. The ironic thing was that Matty bought the frame I made for Judd at my previous fundraising event, and then when Matty was killed, that Judd tribute frame was sitting in Matty's bedroom.

Colin, Matty's dad, said to me, "Josh I want to give you the Judd frame because I know that's what Matt would want—to know that it went to further your recovery."

Colin and I became really close after Matty passed away. We spent so much time together. We trained together at the gym at least three or four times a week. Colin had a massive void in his life after Matty passed away; I had one too. I guess in a way we both helped fill a little bit in each other's lives over time. Of course I would never replace Matty; no one ever could. It was just cool that we were able to spend this time together and it meant so much to me that Colin gave me the frame to auction off so that I could get to Project Walk. At the fundraiser, when the frame went up for auction, I started tearing up because it meant so much to me.

All of a sudden my good mate Hayden Graham called out, "I'll give you 1,000 bucks for it."

That did it for me—I fell apart! I spoke about what the frame meant to me. Then, the bidding took off, but the funny thing was that Hayden was the only one bidding. He was bidding against himself!

He said, "Nah, $1,300... Nah, $1,600," and then he just said, "I want to pay $1,600, I want to buy it for $1,600 but you have to keep it Josh."

I was speechless. I didn't know what to say. That gesture from Hayden meant so much. It was huge for me because of how I felt about that frame and the history and memories it had. The connection of that frame had now come full circle—from me, it passed to Judd, then to Matty, and then back to me through Hayden. It was such an emotional time for me.

Family, friends, and the boys made the fundraiser successful with all their purchases and donations. We raised nearly $20,000 that night.

With the money we raised, and some extra financial support from mum, there was just enough to get Amelia and I to America. We planned the trip and left for Project Walk in September 2011.

# Kay

With the opportunity to go to Project Walk, Josh had the best shot to further his recovery, lose his walking stick, and hopefully improve his gait. His goal was to get the very best of training in a state of the art facility with trainers who were qualified spinal cord injury recovery specialists, and on the cutting edge of activity-based recovery programs. We couldn't wait to get Josh over there and get him started.

Hearing about Project Walk gave the fitness program a whole new meaning for Josh. So in order to begin preparing Josh for the intense training sessions that he would go through while in America, Josh's friend Colin arranged for sponsorship from the Bell Street Gym. He then commenced training Josh four nights a week on weights and strengthening.

Amelia started Josh on a healthier diet, and with Colin's help, she designed an additive program to compliment Josh's training and diet. For the first time in many years, Josh started to bulk up in a healthy way. He was so very strong and fit. He even started going to bed earlier. I had never seen him look so well, and the weight he gained, which was all muscle, made him look amazing! He was so strong and powerful.

In the past, he was a real night owl. Now his life was disciplined and focused on the goals of ditching his walking stick and being as fit as possible before he got to the US in order to allow him to maximize his time at Project Walk.

A house was available for rent near the Project Walk facility in Carlsbad, California. It had four bedrooms, three bathrooms, and a pool. Amelia and Josh could share the house and costs with another two families from Australia who were also attending Project Walk at the same facility. So without any hesitation, it was booked for the six-week period that they would be in Carlsbad.

I was happy that Amelia wanted to travel with Josh. I was only working part time at that stage and couldn't afford to go with him. Amelia was also committed to Project Walk, and it made sense that she went with Josh for the six weeks.

After mum died, and Josh had lost a fourth friend from a motorbike accident, Josh had made a goal to ditch his walking stick, which had been his constant companion for the past nine years. He was committed to a fitness program supported by Simon and the team at Vitality, including Jenny, an acupuncturist. Simon also arranged sponsorship for Josh from the local gym Sweat, which predominantly offered Josh a Cardio workout.

So beginning in August 2010, Josh embarked on a fitness campaign. He had his goal and was determined to achieve it. Hearing about Project Walk gave the fitness program a whole new meaning for Josh.

By the time Josh and Amelia left for America, I could honestly say that I have never seen Josh so fit and committed to achieving the goal to "Ditch the Stick." It was such an exciting time for all of us. I saw the improvements in Josh every day and I was happy that he had the opportunity to improve his gait through the programs offered at Project Walk.

We arrived in Carlsbad and headed straight to the house we rented for the time that we would be attending Project Walk. The brochure did the house far more justice than it deserved. It was disappointing to see that the actual house in which we arrived and went inside certainly didn't match its advertised description. However, I wasn't going to let that take away from the excitement of going to Project Walk and what I was going to achieve there.

Amelia and I quickly grabbed the bedroom that had the most space and had its own private bathroom. It also had stairs that led directly down to the pool, so we wouldn't have to come back through the house. It would do for what we needed.

Now that the home base was sorted, we took the rest of the day to get ourselves familiar with our new surroundings and prepare for our morning meeting at Project Walk. I think all the excitement and possibilities of what I was going to be presented with in the morning had robbed me of a decent night's sleep. Of course that was nothing unusual as the days of getting a decent sleep had been nonexistent since the accident. We made sure that we had a solid breakfast to fuel us for a day of training then we headed off to the facility.

As I went through the doors of Project Walk, it was like going into a different world. I had not ever seen a training facility like this before. I was introduced to my two trainers whose names ironically just happened to be JW and Josh.

I thought, *Well, that's a good start!*

They talked me through their program and exactly what they offered in their training, and right from the start they were so full of encouragement. They didn't waste anytime getting me onto the equipment either, and we pretty much got started right away and I commenced an individually designed training program.

Initially, it was confronting for me to see just how many people were living with a spinal cord injury and to see at what stage they were in their recovery. There were more people in wheelchairs than people with walking aides. It took me some time to process what I saw because other than the mentoring I did with people with spinal cord injuries, this was the first time that I was actually in a facility devoted to people with spinal cord injuries since I had left rehab over 11 years ago.

The extent of injuries that most of the people at Project Walk were dealing with, I hadn't seen since my rehab days in Melbourne. I was overwhelmed with thoughts of my own journey and what I had managed to achieve. I had the notion that perhaps if I hadn't had the drive, determination, and belief to walk, or at least to be at the point of improving and having the movement and mobility I had, then I didn't know where would I be. Would I have even made it to here to Project Walk in Carlsbad? What if I had accepted the prognosis given to me from all my medical team from day one—that I had no hope of recovery, and the "no hope" message they continually drilled into me each day in hospital and the rehab? If I took on board and accepted what they all said to me, then I may never have pushed past through all of it.

I wouldn't be at Project Walk with the opportunity to further my recovery because the medical prognosis would have been it for me. I wouldn't have given any thought to what I might be able to get back, or God forbid, ever walk again! All that would have been gone if I had listened to and accepted what my medical team initially said. I truly think that I would have never survived if I were bedridden or totally dependent on others. It would not have felt right for me. After all, my parents had drilled into me the importance of being independent from when I was a small child!

So I didn't listen and I didn't accept any of it! I chose to follow my recovery through an alternative health path, with some very untraditional practitioners and methods.

I wondered, *How many people with a spinal cord injury in this same situation as me were delivered the same "no hope" messages by the same specialists? How many people didn't know what was possible? When faced with such intense, continual, and negative prognoses, how many people just gave up? How many people had no knowledge of Project Walk? How many people didn't know my message and my journey and what I had managed to achieve?*

The injured people who were in this training facility with me were the exceptions. Like me, these people were looking for answers beyond the ones they had been told. Like me, they believed that recovery was possible.

And I can say that because it obviously didn't end there for them either, because here they were training in this facility that spoke the language that says, "Anything is possible," and "Keep trying, keep at it."

What really impressed me was that if people came into Project Walk in a wheelchair, then all of their training was done out of it! This was a huge psychological benefit! The positivity, the encouragement, and the supportiveness that surged through this centre were all overwhelming for me.

Where I always had to fight for any slither of acknowledgment during my hospital and rehab days, which I never got from any of the medical specialists back home, Project Walk was hundreds of times better. Every time someone achieved something positive, the trainers instantly shouted encouraging words and even high-fived or soft punched the knuckles of the person who was being trained.

On the first day, I was just overwhelmed with thoughts and emotions. I was all over the place and as much as I was so happy to be there, I wanted to get back to the house and just be with Amelia and get off the hamster wheel for a second to sort out my thoughts.

# From Amelia's Journal

### We made it to California!

OMG! We were actually in Carlsbad in California... Project Walk...We made it!

The house we had paid rent for IN ADVANCE! Was a real disappointment...

Note to self: Don't always believe what you see in the beautifully photographed glossy brochure is what you are actually going to get!

The plan was to stay for 6 weeks! And Josh had BIG PLANS to train Monday to Thursday 8am-11am or 9am-12pm at Project Walk.

I had BIG PLANS to ATTEND EVERY session and RECORD EVERY session! This wasn't by any means going to be a holiday!

I was going to be juggling several major 'supporting roles'... Here's the 'role' list-

*The camera lady

*Mentor

*Best friend

*Support system- (you could probably add in counselor/therapist)

*Massage lady- (very important)

*Water lady- (even more important)

*Catheter lady- (the important list is continuing...)

*Life partner/spouse-wife/girlfriend/alpha female- (all round female superstar!)

With all these titles and the amount of work involved, I wondered how I was going to keep my emotions at bay!

After the first day I thought we were about to book our flights back to Australia!!! This was the first time Josh had been back into any rehabilitation centre since the passing of Bronte (the only person who ever understood Josh and what he goes through). It was also extremely confronting for Josh to see how far he had come (from seeing other participants with injuries as severe as his). I was beginning to understand why Josh vowed to never help anyone with a spinal cord injury after Bronte passed away. Especially after all the mentoring Josh went through with Bronte helping him in *his recovery and believing Bronte WOULD recover just like Josh was doing... And then the shock of Bronte passing before he got to recover.*

*I think having the camera there and me filming brought a big dose of reality into the mix for Josh! No footage of Josh was ever captured from when he was at his worst (as he believed if he saw himself he would realize how bad he was and believe he wouldn't recover) this was THE 11 years of reality hitting him from all areas. Josh and I didn't talk for about an hour after leaving Project Walk that day. The reality that he should be in an electric wheelchair with little movement in one arm, the emotions that for 11 years had been put aside to allow only positive energy to heal had all come to the surface AT ONCE! He didn't know how to digest this total confronting, real, emotional cocktail.*

*I didn't know if he was going to cry, scream or punch something and I was very unsure if I could cope with this emotional uncertainty with him for 6 weeks....*

I was actually shocked at my own reaction. I guess when you have the picture in your mind of how something is going to be, and it turns out to be very different to how you thought it was going to be, it just throws you. Don't get me wrong, Project Walk was better than I imagined. It was all the emotions and seeing so many other people living my life that threw me. I wasn't ready for all the doses of reality, especially on my first day.

I'm sure Amelia thought when we left the first day, I was going to go back to the house and pack up and fly back to Melbourne. I barely said two words to her when I came back from Project Walk. I couldn't even properly explain to her what I was thinking and feeling. Even though I tried to explain, there was so much shit going through my head.

I was so glad she was with me. I think that if I had been there on my own, then I wouldn't have been able to handle it. I might have chucked it in and gone home and lost the opportunity of a lifetime to be trained at such an awesome facility.

It could have been the combination of jetlag, the long-distance travel, a bad night's sleep, the build-up of what was coming, and seeing everything

I saw that day at Project Walk that was just all too much. I also dealt with the hard realization of my emotional journey of the past 11 years, everything I experienced from the start of the accident, the negative hospital and rehab phase, and the complications I still experienced.

It was about the amazing breakthroughs, and the movement I got back, the goals I focused on, the unforgiving pain at times, and all the highs and lows that flashed in front of me.

I just wanted to get back to the house and sleep. Maybe by the next morning, things would look different and I would have time to process everything and get a fresher outlook.

## From Amelia's Journal

### Take 2... Project Walk!

Day two at Project Walk was upon us and I was bracing myself for the day ahead. But Josh had turned all of the emotion from day one into positive motivation. He decided to dedicate his training to Bronte, the boys, his Nan and all those who had donated their time and money to get him there. He promised to work his ass off every second that he was there. And he did! Rain, hail or shine, illness or bowel "issues," we were there doing a three hour session, 4 times a week!

He worked so hard and with so much determination I became worried he would burn out!

Not only did he train at Project Walk for three hours in the morning he would also then complete one hour of weight training with me in the gym in the afternoon!

Josh had turned overnight into A TRAINING MONSTER MACHINE!

What a difference a day makes! During day two, I did exactly what I was there to do... Train hard!

I did around three hours at Project Walk. I worked out so much that my trainer Josh eventually told me that I had done enough for one day!

I rang mum and asked her to come over to experience Project Walk with me. She had been through my whole recovery journey and I wanted her to see the programs and the training at Project Walk. I really wanted her to see the results they achieved with SCI people, and especially their positive and encouraging attitude. I also wanted her to see how much I was improving and getting results from being over here.

# Kay

From day one at Project Walk, Josh felt his body waking up. It was so amazing for all of us to observe! I received videos that Amelia sent me and it was unbelievable how much progress he was making. Josh was so excited about his training at Project Walk and he felt that he had a program at last, which given time would give him his life back. While there, Josh worked out four days a week for three hours a day. He and Amelia also joined a local gym to concentrate on weights and further add to Josh's training and recovery. Since the house had a swimming pool, when weather permitted they managed to enjoy a swim after a hard morning at Project Walk.

I arrived at Project Walk two weeks into Josh's training. As I entered Project Walk for the first time, I saw happy families full of hope. It was a very emotional time for me. For the first time in 11 years, I had a real sense of relief and I cried. In fact, I cried a lot of the time I was there. I had this all-encompassing sense of relief. After all these years, we finally had a solution.

After meeting Josh's Lead Trainers, Jason and Josh, and the rest of his team, I was blown away by the enthusiasm of everyone involved. The facility looked like a gym and it felt like a gym.

Everyone was happy, motivated, and committed, and I found to be such a positive environment. The centre was so positive with music pumping, high-fives, laughter, and encouragement; the only difference was that there were people in wheelchairs. There were also some people like Josh who were exercising to improve their gait.

I asked Josh's trainer Jason whether he thought Josh would ever run again, and with no hesitation he answered, "Absolutely."

Jason's confidence amazed me.

Initially Josh was taken aback, because for the last 11 and a half years, we had not been around wheelchairs and other spinal cord injuries. But he worked through it and concentrated on what his trainers told him. Amelia did an amazing job as she filmed Josh and made sure he had plenty of water and ate the right food. It was a real team effort.

I loved my time at Project Walk, and I truly loved staying in Carlsbad at the Best Western Hotel. It was an old hotel but very clean and fresh, the staff was amazing and the location was right on the ocean.

Josh, Amelia, and I set up a daily routine from the start of my time there. They came to the Hotel for breakfast, and while Josh sorted out his daily routine, Amelia and I went for walks along the foreshore. On many occasions, we saw dolphins swimming in the ocean. They were such special and memorable times. On our return, we had breakfast and went to Project Walk.

I was only in Carlsbad for two weeks before I needed to return home to Melbourne. Amelia and Josh kept me up to date with his progress, which even though many of the changes he experienced were very subtle, they were amazing to me and left me full of hope for the possiblities.

Josh kept feeling more of his body waking up and it was so exciting because more movement and agility was returning, and Josh's body was responding to the training so quickly.

On his last day, he rang me in tears. In the last five minutes of his last Project Walk session, Josh ran! The words of Josh's trainer Jason came true. Jason told me that Josh would "absolutely" run one day again, and that day arrived on Josh's last day at Project Walk in the very last minutes of his training.

Josh running was not the end—it was just another step towards achieving his final goal of walking down the street without any assistance and with no one having to wait for him.

What a send off! What a gift it was for Josh to take away with him from the whole Project Walk experience.

I cried and thought to myself, *Thank God we didn't listen to the original prognosis of the medical team and we supported each other, and with our friends we built own recovery program!*

The six weeks that I attended Project Walk just flew by. I experienced the best training by the best trainers, and achieved the best results I could have hoped for. The program my trainers designed for me made my body respond in ways that amazed me.

Right from the beginning, one of my trainers, Jason, said to mum, "Josh will absolutely run one day."

On my last day at Project Walk, in my last five minutes of training, I did just that—I ran! Sure, my first attempt at running after all these years of restricted movement was a little bit awkward, but I still managed to run. It was the most bittersweet moment I experienced in the 11 years since my accident, but it was a defining moment in my recovery and I now had that moment of achievement to bring back home with me. It was time to return home to Melbourne, so I brought all the training techniques, information, and everything that I had learned from the trainers at Project Walk and incorporated it all into my everyday living.

Back in Melbourne, I hit an all-time low. I felt that I had finally found an answer to my recovery in the training programs at Project Walk, but then I had to leave it behind to return home. I suddenly felt like I had no direction and I was struggling to even do any training. I hadn't managed to "ditch the stick" like I planned and even though I wasn't really depressed, I wasn't exactly in good head space either. I had to do something to shift this slump I was in because there were some celebrations coming up that I was really looking forward to.

I started to focus on the good things that were coming up, like my birthday, and of course, my marriage proposal to Amelia. Each day I started to feel a little clearer and more positive. No sooner had I started to turn things around that we were in the month of November and celebrated some important milestones. I had my thirtieth birthday celebration, and of course, my surprise marriage proposal to Amelia, which she accepted with a big yes!

Before we knew it, December arrived and Christmas was coming up. As a Christmas present, mum bought Amelia and I two tickets to Bali. My first trip to Bali was when mum was pregnant with me in 1981. The next time was when I was 12 years old, which was just after mum and dad split up. I continued to visit a few more times before my accident and I enjoyed the fun relaxed lifestyle, the surf, the weather, and the Balinese people. Since my accident, I had been back to Bali three or four times. It was a place I could relax and be comfortable. We have good friends there and they were always very supportive and helpful in introducing me to healers that I knew would further my recovery.

When Amelia and I first arrived, we spent New Year's Eve at our frend Asri's home, which overlooked Jimbaran Bay. Her home was very large and allowed us a lot of privacy. We basically had our own suite downstairs, and it also had a swimming pool where we spent a lot of our time relaxing and enjoying the sun. So for the first week, we enjoyed a quiet time living in a residential area of Bali away from the busy lifestyle of Kuta and Legian.

While staying at Asri's, she introduced us to a healer—a shaman—who she thought would help me with my ongoing recovery.

The first time we met him, Asri translated for me (since he couldn't speak English) that he said to her, "I don't know what's happened to this man, but his body is like shards of broken crystal."

He then motioned for me to walk so he could see how I moved.

## Kay

Our recovery program for Josh had included alternative methods and healers right from the morning after the accident and Bali was just an extension of that. I knew that Josh could further his recovery with healers who also brought the mind-body-spirit-healing-recovery process to a new level of experience. Over time, Bali introduced an extended number to our recovery team. We were not restricted by what was impossible, so we were open to new ideas and different healers.

Josh worked with this one particular healer that my friend Asri introduced us to the first week Josh and Amelia arrived in Bali—he was a Timorese shaman. Watching this healer work on Josh was scary and quite confronting at times. I was really nervous about some of the movements and adjustments he did to Josh. They seemed so intense that sometimes it got too much and I had to leave the room. I didn't want Josh to see my tears, but I trusted that Josh knew what he was doing. The more concerned I was, the more Josh said, "Bring it on."

The first thing the healer said in Indonesian to Asri was, "I don't know what has happened to this man, but his inner body is that of Broken Crystal Shards," and then his next comment about Josh was, "Whoever had operated on his right leg had not reattached the right hip flexor muscle properly. The muscle has been sown on backwards."

The amazing thing about that last statement was that there was nothing to indicate Josh had been operated on his leg. This healer determined all this information from only observing Josh walking, because at that stage, he had not yet spoken to Josh or asked any questions about Josh's body.

The shaman's comment was interesting to me because, going back to when Josh was operated on three days after his accident, later that day, Josh said something really strange even though Josh could not feel anything below his neck because he was totally paralyzed.

"They have done something to the muscle at the top of my right leg that was operated on. My leg feels empty."

I said, "You must be imagining things. You can't feel it."

Josh just repeated, "It is empty. They have made a mistake."

His right leg never really communicated with his body for several years, and this healer picked that up just by observing Josh walk.

I thought he was very talented and very intuitive to Josh's body.

This healer surprised me with how much information he picked up just by watching me walk. He actually blew me away with what he said about my right leg, because from the moment I woke up from my operation four days after my accident, I knew there was something wrong with my right leg. It felt empty.

No matter whom we asked, they all said the same thing, "Everything was done to procedure in the operation."

This healer didn't even ask me any questions about my operation or recovery, yet he knew what went wrong. I trusted everything he said, and I was happy for him to work on me. I always carry my MRIs in my iPhone in case something goes wrong. We set up the laptop and—surprise, surprise—he got it! He really understood the body's pathways.

I had several sessions with him. He worked on me for one or two hours once a week, sometimes twice a week, and the sessions were grueling. I thought he was going to massage me like the other masseurs did, but his technique was very different to theirs. It was very intense!

Sometimes his work got so full on that Amelia and Mum left the room in tears. At times it was so painful, but I could feel my body respond to what he was doing.

Once towards the end of one session, my body was painless and relaxed. This was the first time in 12 years that I had been pain free and this relaxed. It only lasted a minute but it was such an amazing feeling.

He worked with spirit also, and sometimes he seemed to either come across some blockage in me, or in himself, and he would stop for a moment, pray, and seemed to have a conversation. Then, he would start working on me again.

Mum and Amelia filmed a lot of his healing work. He was okay with that but would not let them film while he was praying.

For the last two weeks of our stay in Bali, mum booked Amelia and I into a hotel in Kuta. We stayed at the new Pullman Hotel on the beach between Kuta and Legian.

The week before we left Bali, I went down to breakfast and had my usual bacon and eggs. The minute I bit into the bacon I said to Amelia it was off and within a few hours I was so sick. In fact, Amelia had to get a doctor in and I ended up on a drip for 24 hours. I was too weak to have any further sessions with the shaman. Physically and mentally, I could not have stood the pain, so I never went back to him for my last two sessions. It took all my strength through the following week just to get well enough to fly home.

When we arrived home to Melbourne, we easily paced back into our normal lifestyle. We were back in our apartment in Port Melbourne, and it was summer so I enjoyed the good weather and the slower pace of the city and life in general.

Throughout the summer months, Amelia and I initially didn't do a lot of work with our training. We did a couple of sessions now and then but no specific programs. I would to go the gym and work the pushbike for 20 minutes and do some weights. There wasn't any hardcore training like I did in Project Walk; it was just enough to keep me moving forward.

After years of doing some sort of training most days, I think I was just going through the motions then. It felt a bit like being on autopilot. Each day was no different from the other; I didn't introduce any new programs or change my training, and I think I just got too comfortable and a bit complacent.

I felt I was a bit lost after Project Walk. I felt something was wrong.

I didn't feel I had a set direction or determined goal. I didn't really feel like I was me anymore, and I felt like I wasn't running my own body. I wasn't connecting in the way I had been. Something shifted within me but I didn't understand what it was. This shift started to affect my sleeping pattern and I didn't sleep well at all.

Sleeping was difficult since my accident and proper rest was pretty much non-existent for me.

Even when I did manage to sleep, it was never a good night's rest because I spent most of my time tossing and turning to get comfortable. I cannot sleep naturally like other people do. I actually physically wake up and have to sit up and move to the other side of the bed, then roll over because my body doesn't turn as naturally as able-bodied peoples' do.

I was prescribed Xanax tablets on and off throughout my recovery to relax my body, and since my sleep pattern was so interrupted, I started to take one at night to help me relax and sleep. For the first time in 11 years, I had a completely restful night's sleep. I woke up with energy and I felt good. I think I got six to eight hours of solid sleep. For the first time in months, my body relaxed and had a break and it was great. I woke up feeling fine and very rested.

I thought, Sweet, *I can just pop a pill.*

And I knew that when I went to bed, I would have an amazing night's sleep. My body was going to be able to have a rest and I was not going to feel pain and toss and turn all night.

A few months went by, and I realized I used the Xanax to help me sleep every single night. In the six months leading up to January 2012, the dosages became stronger because I developed more of an immunity to it, but because I didn't feel any side effects, and I had these great sleeps, I didn't think anything of it.

By the end of February 2012, I started getting little migraines. I had them two or three times a week when I previously had migraines probably once or twice a year. I started to worry a bit and I became concerned with the frequency and intensity of them, so I began to visit my chiropractor Simon every time they came on. He did some adjustments and the migraine would go away. However, while the adjustments gave me relief, they didn't solve the problem, and the migraines became more and more frequent and became harder to cope with. The intensity and frequency of them got to the point where I just threw up and then slept the rest of it off for three or four hours. With all the different things I went through with my accident, although I had some concerns about them, I dismissed them by thinking it was only a stage I was going through, and eventually it would all settle down at some point.

I was about to be proven very wrong.

My car was due to be serviced. I phoned mum to organize for her to come over in the morning, follow me to the mechanic's workshop to drop my car off, and then she would drive me back to my place.

That morning, I woke up with the same kind of throbbing migraine that I had become so used to. When I called mum that morning to double check that she was still coming over to follow me to the mechanic's workshop, I didn't tell her that I was having one my usual migraines. Amelia offered to stay home from work and look after me but I told her I was fine and that she should go to work. But, by the time mum got to my place, the migraine was getting worse.

I said to mum, "You are going to have to get me to Simon's for an adjustment."

Mum practically had to carry me to her car. Even she was getting concerned at this stage.

By the time we arrived at Simon's practice, I couldn't move anything. My left side was completely numb and it felt really heavy. I felt totally paralyzed. I became so immobilized that Simon and one of his other chiropractors had to physically carry me into his clinic.

He worked on me for about 20 minutes. My acupuncturist James also came down to the clinic to work on me in between Simon working on other people, so that he could get some of my acupuncture points stimulated and to respond, but nothing was working.

Normally, these healings worked on me immediately and I would be fine. But that day, nothing worked. My body did not respond to anything Simon and James did, and I just got worse and worse by the minute.

Finally Simon said to mum, "I think Josh is having a stroke, and I don't think you have time to get an ambulance. I think you have get him straight to hospital."

Simon thought that if it wasn't a stroke that was causing this sudden paralysis that my body was experiencing, then the plate in my neck might have moved, and that could also be the cause of the problem. So they put a neck brace on my neck to keep that area stabilized enough for me to be safely and comfortably transported to hospital.

They carried me back out of his practice and put me in mum's car, and she took me straight to the emergency hospital.

## Kay

I arrived at Josh's early so that we had time to talk and catch up, but he was still in bed with a migraine and not showing any signs of getting better. In fact he was getting worse by the minute.

I started to get really nervous, so I rang Simon and somehow dragged and pulled Josh into the car. By time I got to Simon's practice, I wasn't able to get Josh out of my car, so Simon and one of his chiro team members came out and carried Josh in. I became more and more scared. Nothing was working!

I thought, *What the hell! Oh how I hate this injury—just when everything is going well for Josh something like this happens!"*

I asked Simon if I should take Josh to the Epworth (our emergency hospital), but Simon said he wanted to work on Josh a little more.

Nothing was working—the adjustments, the acupuncture—I was really scared now!

Josh had had his neck adjusted in Bali by the shaman. Simon thought the plate may have been loosened in his neck, or that Josh was actually have a stroke since he was becoming incoherent! I wanted to call an ambulance, but Simon thought I should take him straight to the Epworth.

I don't know what I was thinking in agreeing to this but I was just so scared! As we sped across the city, I called Amelia and told her Josh was worse. He could no longer feel his left side and his body was shutting down.

For the first time since the accident, I prayed that if Josh was having a stroke and was going to face paralysis once again, then I wanted him to die. I loved him too much to want him to have to go through all of this again. I was not giving up on him—it was just that I had seen him suffer through so much because of his initial injury that I truly loved him too much for him to have to suffer through recovery again from scratch.

When we arrived at the Epworth hospital, I bolted into emergency and pleaded for help. They didn't have any staff available, so they said he would have to walk in. I asked them where the wheelchairs were, and somehow I had to get him into a chair.

Finally, an orderly arrived, and between us we were able to get Josh from my car into the chair and into emergency.

I had a quick examination once mum and an orderly got me into emergency at the hospital. The admitting doctor was concerned that my plate might have moved, so he wanted the opinion of an orthopedic surgeon before doing anything more with me. With everything that was happening to me, my body was exhausted. I was just so tired that right after all the tests were done, I went to sleep.

When I woke up, I felt a neck brace on me. My arms were beneath the sheets so I couldn't actually see anything. Then, I saw I was in hospital in the emergency room.

I completely freaked out! I thought the last twelve years were all a lie!

Here I was in hospital in emergency with a neck brace on and sheets covering me from my shoulders down.

I thought, *What the hell is going on?*

Just as I was about to completely lose it, Amelia and mum walked in the room. I just started crying because as soon as I saw Amelia walk in, I realized that I was still in the present time and that my mind was only playing tricks on me.

I struggled to understand what was happening to me and why my body had shut down to the point of being totally paralyzed again. A massive fear came over me.

I was as fit as I had ever been. I was training really hard. I was training regularly with Colin and also training by myself. I no longer drank alcohol, I really looked after myself, I had proper rest and sleep and the food I ate was much healthier. Realistically, I thought I was really fit, but there I was, with my body closing down, and I didn't know what the hell was going on.

I was so scared, and so were Amelia and mum.

I said to Amelia, "If you want to leave and just get on with your life then I will understand."

And I meant that. I would have understood if she decided that this was too much, or too hard, and chose to say no to it—but she didn't. She just said that she would be here with me to get me through this.

My personal orthopedic surgeon wasn't available, so the hospital called in the orthopedic surgeon who was on duty. He came in, and explained that they were going to do a CAT Scan and MRIs to identify the cause of this paralysis.

We had to wait several hours before we got the results. It was so scary.

I just kept thinking, *I am back to where I was 12 years ago.*

Finally, the results came back to us. Thank goodness it was only a severe migraine. It's a funny feeling to be grateful for a severe migraine, but compared to what it could have been, I'll take the migraine any time!

While I was still in massive pain, but at least I knew I would be okay. A nurse came in and gave me a sedative and I went to sleep.

I continued to take the Xanax tablets to help me relax and sleep. I didn't think they were doing me any harm. I didn't experience any side effects, but I decided to decrease the dosage.

Over the years, I preferred not to take prescription drugs unless they were totally necessary. I just felt that it was time to stop relying on Xanax to get me into a proper rest and sleep routine.

It was time to regain focus, reintroduce all the techniques I learned from my alternative recovery team, pick up the pace from this point on, and get my body back into my routine. After being discharged from hospital, I returned to my focused routine and everything was back to normal. I felt fine; I trained, ate healthy, and had quality sleep.

After returning from Project Walk, even my bladder's function improved and I was able to go to the toilet without having to use a catheter. For years I had been intermittently using a catheter because I lost the function that allowed me to release the valve to pee properly, even though I could tell when my bladder was full.

It was fantastic to finally be free from those issues.

After a few weeks, I started to experience problems with my bladder again. It started to get really difficult to pee so I went back to using the catheter, but then I couldn't track it. I couldn't actually get the catheter into my bladder.

It felt like the gap in my urethra was really tight, so I called my doctor who immediately booked me in to see an urologist. After giving me a thorough examination, he scheduled me for surgery the next day.

## The background to my bladder issues

It was many years since I had issues using a catheter. About six years prior to this surgery, I was at a friend's place and I decided to stay the night. I must have fallen asleep on my catheter, which was in my pocket, and I bent it. When I woke up and went to go the toilet, I realized the catheter was damaged, but it was the only one I had with me.

I was about two hours away from my home, so going home to pick up another one was not an option. I had to use the bent one I had with me. As I tracked the catheter into my bladder, the catheter turned inside my urethra and it got stuck. When I pulled it out, I tore the side of my urethra, which made a massive hole in it. There was blood going everywhere, and it was so bad that the blood actually bubbled out of my pants.

I jumped in my car and started to drive to the hospital. My Aunty Susie worked at Frankston hospital, which was the closest hospital from my mate's place where I stayed overnight.

I thought, *I've just got to make it to emergency.*

I felt faint and light headed and I began to lose consciousness, but I kept going because I knew I was close to the hospital. By the time I got there I was pretty bad. I had lost so much blood that it actually turned black.

I drove myself straight into the emergency entrance of the hospital and parked my car. My Aunty Susie was waiting for my arrival at the emergency entrance with a wheelchair and blanket. She notified the emergency team that I was coming, so when I arrived, she helped me into a wheelchair and got me inside where the emergency team quickly stabilized me, stopped the bleeding, and cleaned me up.

They told me that they would most likely have to do an in-dwelling catheter straight through the side of my stomach, which meant I would have to wear a catheter bag connected on the outside of my stomach for the rest of my life.

I was absolutely adamant that there was no way that was going to happen! I didn't want them to stop until they could get the catheter into my bladder the right way.

It took them about an hour to track the catheter back into my bladder. Through all the discomfort and pain I went through at that time, it was worth it, because they managed to track the catheter back into my urethra. They kept me in hospital overnight, and in the morning when I felt strong enough, I was discharged and I drove home very carefully so as not to disturb anything.

This all related to the present bladder problem I was experiencing. What I was unaware of was that because of the damage I did to my urethra by pulling out the bent catheter, there was scar tissue that started forming around that damaged area of my urethra. I was totally unaware of any potential problems because after I returned from Project Walk, I went through a long period of time where I was able to pee normally.

After all these years, and especially for those few months after I returned from Project Walk, I peed whenever I wanted. I didn't have to use a catheter and it was great! But then there I was, back in hospital, and I was being prepped for surgery that would hopefully remove the scar tissue.

When the surgeon went in, he saw the scar tissue had grown so badly that it squashed my urethra. It became so hard that the catheter couldn't actually track past it anymore. The surgeon delicately removed the scar tissue. Since I was used to using the catheter, the surgeon left it in overnight and removed it the next day.

Within two weeks of the surgery, I felt my urethra close up again. Initially, I wasn't aware that this happened. I just thought I was having one of those moments that it was hard to track the catheter, and because I had these issues so many times before, I didn't think anything was wrong.

My car still needed to be serviced, so I booked my car with a mechanic near Hastings where my mate Toddy lived. I drove down early to hang out with Toddy at his place. Toddy and I chilled for a bit that night. We watched some television and had a few Hennessys and a couple of beers. As time went on, I decided to stay the night and take my car into the garage in the morning.

I went to sleep in Toddy's spare room. Every time I lay down on the bed, I felt like I was going to pee, so I would quickly get up and go to the toilet. I couldn't track the catheter since it started giving me problems the night before, and now I couldn't actually get the catheter back into my bladder. I ran out of lubricant and I didn't even have a spare tube of it with me.

I sat on the toilet and tried to pee normally but I couldn't release my bladder, so I went and lay down again. As soon as I did, I felt like I was going to pee myself. I probably repeated this cycle about 20 times throughout the night as I went backwards and forwards to the toilet and attempted to pee.

By the time morning came, I was so dehydrated and I didn't get any sleep. I was too scared to have a Xanax because I thought that I would either have another Dysreflexia episode and not wake up, or that I would piss the bed. The fact that I didn't take Xanax that night played a huge role. I basically went cold turkey on using the tablets. It was not until later on that I realized how significantly my body depended on Xanax.

I probably only had half an hour of sleep that night. Initially, I didn't feel too bad, but I did feel really tired. Toddy was already up and was playing with his young son. I helped Toddy prepare some food for him.

All of a sudden, I started getting jolts in my brain, which felt like I was getting electrocuted. It felt like my brain went *zap* and then jolts would follow.

I said to Toddy, "I don't feel that good. I think I need some water."

I had another jolt. I felt like my body was electrocuted! My body sort of shook for a second and it felt like my brain just stopped, but then it rebooted itself, and my body locked up.

I started to get really concerned.

I thought, *What the fuck is going on with me?*

I had never experienced anything like this problem before. I went outside to get some air. I walked to my car to get something out of it. As I got into my car, I had such a big jolt that actually threw me off my feet and I landed into the car's back seat. I took a breather and tried to settle myself down.

Then I went back inside the house and said to Toddy, "I'm not good. There's something wrong."

It was 8 a.m. and I rang mum.

I said to her, "I've got to get my car fixed. Can you come down and pick me up so I don't have to worry about sitting around all day?"

She said she would come straight down. It would take her about an hour to drive from her home in Port Melbourne to Toddy's house in Hastings.

While mum was on her way, Toddy went to the shops to buy some food and a bottle of Powerade for me. I thought that I had dehydrated myself so much and that was why my body was getting these jolts. What I needed was some solid food and electrolytes, so hopefully this would replenish me and settle my body down.

Toddy quickly returned with the food and electrolytes. I sat down with him and started to eat and drink, but then I had another major jolt. It was so strong that I threw my burger back onto my plate.

I would feel fine but then I would get a massive zap in my brain, and everything would lock up, and I would miss two seconds of time. This cycle of my body jolting and then feeling fine kept repeating, so Toddy took me outside to get some fresh air.

I drank a litre and a half of water to try to rehydrate myself.

I walked around Toddy's backyard, but then the next thing I knew, I was on the ground. I had such a big jolt that it threw me off my feet and I slid on the grass right in front of Toddy. By this stage he was completely freaked out! Neither of us knew what was happening. This had never happened to me before, and I was scared shitless.

Toddy helped me up and took me back inside. At that moment, mum arrived. She sat down and was about to drink her cup of coffee. I said to mum that we needed to leave straight away and to forget the coffee because I just wanted to go home. I wanted to lie down and go to sleep. Mum said she would be quick and to relax for a minute.

As mum and Toddy talked, she looked at me and said, "Josh, you just don't look good mate. There's more happening here than just dehydration."

I was about to answer her but I lost consciousness. I blacked out, and I don't remember a thing after that.

The next time I woke up, mum and Toddy were on their knees next to me and the ambulance medics were coming through the door.

# Kay

I arrived at Toddy's home and went inside. I was about to sit down and have a cup of coffee when I noticed Josh didn't look right.

He was really impatient with me and he wanted to leave immediately. After the long drive so early in the morning, I felt really tired. I just wanted to have a quick coffee before we left.

We were both sitting on bar stools next to each other when Josh had a massive jolt.

I said to him, "There's more going on here than dehydration."

Josh threw his head back at that moment and at first I thought that he was messing with me because he was always trying to scare me. Then I realized his eyes had rolled back into his head and he was rigid.

I screamed to Toddy!

It only lasted for seconds, but we both grabbed him and got him to the floor into the recovery position.

Then he started to choke. There was nothing that Toddy and I could use to get his mouth open, so we both just forced his mouth open with our hands. He seemed to relax for a moment, and we did what everyone says not to do—we put our fingers in his mouth to release his tongue.

Then, bang! My thumb and Toddy's finger were both trapped in Josh's mouth.

He bit down so hard that I thought, There goes my thumb.

We tried to remain calm and release our fingers at the same time.

Finally, we managed to pry our fingers out of his grip. Toddy's wife called the ambulance while this was all happening. There was blood everywhere from Josh's tongue and from our fingers.

I remained calm outwardly but on the inside I was terrified! I could not believe what was happening. I silently repeated to myself how much I hated this injury and I prayed that Josh would be okay. I wondered how much more my son had to endure from this vengeful, cruel injury.

Toddy and I held Josh tightly and spoke to him quietly in an attempt to keep him calm. The medics arrived as Josh started to regain consciousness. Josh didn't know what had happened. We didn't want to scare him so we just told him that he fell off the stool.

The medics quickly stabilized him. Since Josh had been booked in for further surgery the next day, I asked the ambulance to transport him to the Epworth. I was so glad that I had waited to have the coffee. If we were in the car when that happened, I don't know what I would have done because I wasn't familiar with the area and it was so far from home.

We were later told that the seizure was so powerful that if Josh were on his own or in his car when it happened, then he would have died!

I followed the ambulance to the hospital. There I was, calling Amelia yet again, and telling her more distressing news about Josh. We arranged for her to meet us at Epworth.

Poor Amelia had to deal with yet another hospital trip, and they weren't even married yet, so I said to her, "I think you're getting 'the worse' before you get married."

Then I rang Josh's father and we arranged to meet him at Epworth as well.

As I sat in the car while I was driving back to Melbourne, I was so confused, frustrated, and sad. I wondered what would happen next and when Josh would finally get a break from all of this. He had tried so hard, but then this happened out of nowhere.

For the first time since his accident, I seriously felt like my confidence in his recovery was totally destroyed.

I completely blacked out for 10 or 15 minutes. By the time I woke up, the ambulance was already at Toddy's house and the medics were coming through the door. I saw that there was blood everywhere, and I didn't know what the hell had happened. There was blood on my face and even all over mum's hand.

I found out later on that I actually had a seizure. I apparently started to choke, and mum and Toddy tried to open my mouth to clear my airways while I was on my side, but I bit down on mum's thumb right down to the bone. My jaw completely locked up. When I woke up, my jaw was killing me and I couldn't move it.

At that stage we didn't know what was going on, but because I was already booked into Epworth Hospital to have my surgery the next day, the ambulance took me straight there.

It felt like a terrible worst déjà vu scenario. I was back in an ambulance going to hospital yet again. That was my third trip to hospital within a month, and it was scary because none of this should have been happening! I was as fit and as focused as I had ever been. I felt like my body was finally giving up after all those years of pushing my body beyond its limits. I thought that this was the end and that all my hard work was starting to depreciate because my body just had enough.

In the ambulance on the way to Epworth hospital, I started to think about Xanax and I realized that I hadn't taken a tablet that past night in order to sleep. I thought that I was maybe having a reaction because my body had become so used to taking it. Maybe I was having withdrawal symptoms.

The medics did a great job in rehydrating and stabilizing me after the seizure. When I arrived at the hospital, I was sore and bloodied; my tongue was swollen from me biting on it. I just felt so frustrated, exhausted, and really confused.

Amelia and mum came in to be with me and I wondered about Amelia's commitment to me.

I thought, *What is she thinking? What is she feeling? This has to be taking a toll on her as well. Does she really understand what she has signed up for?*

Everything had been going so well, but then we went through these past two months of hell. I didn't know what the outcome of any of it was going to be. I was too scared to even think about it!

Again, I told Amelia that I wouldn't be surprised if she said that she'd had enough and she wanted to leave me. And again, she said she didn't! She was just so incredibly committed to our future together.

I can't even describe how happy I was when she said that. I loved her so much, and I hated having to watch her watch me go through this shit, but since she was so committed to us getting through it together, I knew that we would be fine.

The medical team at Epworth did brain scans and MRIs on my neck to see whether any of my bones were pressing on my spinal cord, or whether there was any movement in my neck or along my spinal column. I thought there would be some physical explanation as to why I had these migraines and the severe jolts going through my body.

The results came back that I was 100 percent fine! Even though I was happy about this, it made me even more frightened to be on my own because the doctors couldn't give an explanation as to why this was happening and whether or not it would to continue to affect me.

They were confident I didn't have a brain tumour, so I was treated as though I had a massive seizure. With the information the doctors received from asking mum and Toddy about what happened, the doctors were confident it was just a one-off event.

The operation on my urethra went ahead the next day as scheduled. This time, when they removed the scar tissue, something went wrong and the urethra was torn further.

I just seriously could not believe that all this shit was happening to me. I wondered if I would ever get a break.

The specialist team, who had learned from the first operation, left the catheter in for two weeks. While I hated this, the alternative was worse, so I just accepted that it had to be this way.

I came out of recovery much quicker this time, and Amelia and mum were there waiting for me. I was starving so I asked mum to go get me McDonald's.

When I came home from the hospital, my confidence was completely ruined. I spent the next three months recuperating at home. This was a new health crisis that I had to contend with. Since the doctors couldn't explain it, I started to think that maybe my body was finally reacting to the Xanax tablets and it didn't like having the tablets in my system.

Once again, I started addressing my food and water intake. I planned to only eat healthy foods. While I could change and improve my food, I couldn't change or improve my fear of what was happening to me. My uncertainty about my health affected me mentally and emotionally, and it was much worse than what I experienced before.

I did not leave the house unless I was with Amelia. This put more pressure on Amelia because she couldn't do anything or plan to go anywhere, because I didn't know what would happen if I was left by myself. As difficult and as uncertain as it was, I just had to push forward and think of ways about how I could get better.

No one had answers for me, so I retreated back to how I used to think about my health situations and what I used to do when I originally had my accident. I went back to drinking as much pure water as I could. I kept myself fit; I only consumed healthy foods and I made sure I ate at certain times so that my body was always nourished. I would get a jolt as soon as my body was hungry. I was shit scared when I had these jolts, because I didn't know when they were coming or how severe they would be. The felt like my brain was being electrocuted, and my body reacted to them with massive jumps.

For the first time, I was at a loss for how to help myself.

One day I finally got the courage to go and do something with my friends for the first time in months. I went to my favorite Greek restaurant with Zayne and Tommy. This was something we did regularly and I thought it was going to be great to catch up with the boys.

Since my seizure, I was living like such a hermit. I hadn't seen any of the boys for a while. I didn't want them to see that I wasn't well. I didn't want to worry them that something was wrong, so I kept making excuses not to see them.

After a while when I had used up every possible valid excuse, I thought, *Is this what my life is going to be like? Am I too scared to see my mates and too scared to walk out my front door?*

I knew that I wasn't going to live my life like that, so I arranged to catch up with the boys.

I met them at the restaurant, but then half-way through dinner I got another bloody migraine. I couldn't believe that my first time going out with the boys in so long and it was turning out like this.

I had to get out of the restaurant setting, so I drove back to Amelia's work. I blacked out while I was driving so I nearly crashed my car! However, I managed to make it to her work and she took me straight home.

That was it for me! I was too completely scared to do anything. I was too scared to go out or do anything without mum or Amelia with me. My armour had been chinked much worse than it had ever been before my initial accident. Even going through the whole hospital and rehab experience didn't compare with how scared I was now.

I felt like I had no control over my body. I couldn't predict what would happen or when anything would happen. Some days I would be fine and feel like I was starting to get better, but then, *boom!* My body would drop off again or I would experience more jolts.

I constantly drank water. I was too scared to drink anything less than three litres of water each day, or else the jolts would be inevitable.

I tried to figure out what I was going to do with my body. Mentally, I was tested in every way, and I had had many more medical tests done this time than in any other time throughout of the whole 12 years of my injury. It scared the living shit out me!

I felt like I had no control over my body or my thoughts. I couldn't sleep properly and I had migraines all the time. At least if I had a Xanax, then the migraines allowed me to sleep at night.

The problem was that I still had a job to do. I was booked to speak to a number of insurance groups around Australia. I also had a few more talks to do before I returned to Project Walk in California, so before I left Australia, I knew I had to be better.

I became a complete hermit. I just stayed at home. I was even too scared to go training. I'm not someone who easily gets scared about things like this, but I was terrified about what else could happen to me. My life was in lockdown and I didn't understand what the hell was going on with my body or how I could fix it.

I thought I was going to drop off any day and that was going to be the end of me. But, I knew I had to get ready for Project Walk. I was going to be there for four months. This combined with the travel I needed to do with my talks made me focus on getting over my health setbacks.

My biggest motivator to get on top of all my health issues was my marriage to Amelia, which was coming up in February 2012. I wasn't about to let her down with me getting sick again. I had already made the commitment to ditch the stick and walk down the aisle without it. No migraines and other health issues were going to stop me from that.

So I focused on some specific goals, which were amongst the most important goals I ever set and focused upon:

- To wean myself off Xanax so I didn't need to rely on them to help me relax and get a good night's sleep.
- To be well enough and strong enough to return to Project Walk for a four-month timeframe.
- To walk down the aisle at my wedding to Amelia without my stick.

These were my most important goals to achieve.

I wasn't finished with my recovery. This was only the next phase of it. I wasn't going to let go of 12 years of hard work! Not then! Not now! Not ever!

# Chapter 7

# Woody Breaks The Stick!

## Letting go of all the layers...

The past few months had taken a real toll on my body—the migraines, the jolts that made me feel like my body was electrocuted, the fear of knowing they could happen at any time, and the fear of not knowing how the hell I would stop them.

I didn't know what my body was going to do at any given time, and it was really scary, not just for me, but also for Amelia and mum.

Somehow I managed to get through my speaking commitments and they actually went really well. I was fine with the interstate travel that I did in order to get to the places I was going to speaking at. I managed to get through my obligations without any serious health issues.

I still was not comfortable being on my own; I needed to have either Amelia or mum with me all the time. Not knowing what caused these jolts and migraines was what worried me the most.

I had to keep up my training, and focus upon getting better, because my date to return to America to do further recovery work at Project Walk was fast approaching. This time, I was going to stay for four months in order to to give myself the best opportunity to consistently train, and put a real effort in to get more movement and function back.

Mum had gone to America in early June to establish a base for us and start her role at Project Walk. She had found an apartment near the beach in Carlsbad and with the weather being hot there, both Amelia and I were looking forward to beach weather.

The next couple of months flew by and it was now time to return to Project Walk! The first week that Amelia and I returned to California, I caught up with my mate Maddo (Robbie Maddison). He had a BBQ at his house with some of the other boys he rides with. I was in Temecula, which wasn't too far from Maddo's place; I had bought a truck nearby and I stopped by to say, "G'day," to Maddo.

It was a perfect hot sunny day in California.

Maddo just had a new pool built in his backyard and he said to me, "Come for a swim."

I was too scared to be out in the full heat of the sun in case my body reacted and I had one of those jolts. So instead I made my excuses and I stayed in the shade instead. I wasn't being my usual social self. I was so withdrawn from everyone, and I'm sure they wondered what the hell was going on with me. I didn't tell any of them what was really going on. It was too hard to explain to my friends because I didn't even know what was happening myself.

Usually, I would always be the first one in the water and the first one out in the sun. I was a real sun person; I loved the summer months. However, I was so concerned with my health that day, and Maddo must have seen that something wasn't right with me. As we chatted, he told me about a therapist he saw who had been doing some healing work on him. She lived in Encinitas, which wasn't far from Carlsbad. Her name was Uschi and she was a Cranial Sacral therapist.

Uschi helped Maddo with all his injuries from the accidents he sustained from motor cross. Maddo swore by her technique and said he had never received such awesome results. After hearing how impressed Maddo was with Uschi's work, I thought I had nothing to lose by going along to see her myself to see if she could help me with my recovery.

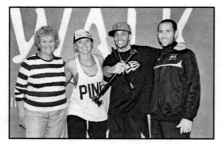

Within just the first week of Uschi working on me, I felt major differences in my body. I called her Golden Fingers because when she touched me, it felt like my whole body responded. I could actually feel my body rejuvenating. Sometimes she didn't even touch me or make physical contact with my body. She would place her hands above me and hover them just above my skin, and I could feel the energy coming out of her hands. When she would move her hands over my back, I could feel my spinal cord fluid pumping through my neck. It felt like my body was trying to open up again, and my mind began to relax. It was such a great healing method.

Uschi worked over my whole body in each session. She started from my pelvic area, slowly worked up to the top of my head, came back down along my arms, and then along my legs to my feet. She only was the most hands-on was when she worked on my neck. She gently pressed on certain pressure points all along my neck. This instantly released pressure in my neck and I just felt my whole neck relax and open up.

I went into the deepest sleeps; it felt like I was on another planet. I didn't know where I went half the time. All I knew was that it was so nice and peaceful.

I had regular sessions with Uschi for a few weeks. I felt great and was doing so much better. I decided to just kick back, take Amelia up to Huntington Beach, and go to a favourite place of ours called Dukes. I had a couple of beers and straight away, I started to feel off, so I stopped drinking the beer and started drinking as much water as was possible.

The work that Uschi did really cleansed my body, so as soon as I put any alcohol in my system, my body reacted to it. I had to keep my body as clean as possible during this cleansing work.

I saw Uschi once or twice a week for a couple of hours at a time. My body responded very well with all the work she did on me. Uschi knew just what my body needed and how to fix my problems, and the jolts and bladder issues ceased. It was just the best result! My body had such great results with her work that I regained my confidence. I felt strong again. I felt like I was becoming Josh again, instead of the scared person I was for the last six months.

I also started my programs at Project Walk again. While I was at Project Walk, one very important thing that they taught me was that it isn't just about walking, but it's about using my body to do whatever I could in order to get it to move.

One day, my trainer Josh and I were messing around by doing some off-the-wall stuff, and training like we did every other day, and I tried to jump. I had tried jumping a couple of times at home a few years after my accident without any success. The problem with me doing any sort of jump is that my right leg either jolts or it goes in the opposite direction while my left leg goes up the right way. I had no coordination in keeping my legs in sync with each other.

We decided to work on my jumping skills and we pulled out the training ladder, which has mini pipes running along material so it unravels into a long ladder that lies on the ground. Josh stood on one side of me to catch me, and I had a physio bench on the other side of me if I went the opposite way. He broke down the action and sequence of how to jump, and I went through it in my head and stood there for a second as I visualized it. In my mind, I actually went back to what it was like to jump in my old snowboarding days. I also thought about being on the motor cross bike, when I would push down the pegs to preload before I jumped.

I tried to remember what it was like to naturally jump without any sports aspect. It was a little bit more difficult to remember, but once I visualized it, I made myself believe that I could do it. Then, I took a jump and I somehow landed it right in the next square.

I couldn't believe it! Both of my feet hit the ground at the same time. I didn't bend my knee out, I didn't fall to the side, and I actually landed on both feet pretty solidly. Well, not very solidly, but solid enough for me!

Then after that, I tried to jump and reach each additional square. I kept perfecting my new skill. I kept getting further and further out, and after a couple of attempts, I ended up making it all the way down the length of the ladder. It was great because it was something my body hadn't done in about 13 years, and it just proved yet again that the body can move forward and continue to recover even 13 years after an injury, and most importantly, it can still learn new things.

While I was in California, one of my best mates, Joshy Cachia, was there at the same time. He was racing for an Australian race team in the American West Coast Super Cross. He trained about 45 minutes away from where I was based, so he came down to Project Walk one time to watch me train. He told me he surfed in his spare time in between training, and racing. He and the boys from his racing team were surfing at Oceanside Beach not far from Project Walk.

Carlsbad and Oceanside beaches were where all the boys went surfing. When I drove along the coast each day, there were always so many people surfing at those awesome coastal beaches. It got me thinking about when I used to surf in Bali before I had my accident.

Joshy asked me if I wanted to come down and watch the boys surf, so we headed off the beach. Over the years since my accident, I watched many people surf so many times, and I really never took much notice of it. Then when I watched Joshy surf, I became really interested in it again.

This day there were actually some dolphins out there surfing the same wave as Joshy. I thought that was amazing. I suddenly had this burning desire to get out there and enjoy doing something that I loved to do in the past.

I told Joshy that I wanted to go surfing with him and the boys, and he said, "Yeah, let's get straight out there."

Life in Carlsbad was so busy that it took about two weeks before we finally organized a day to go down to the beach to join the boys for a surf. Karl, Ash, Joshy, and Jason were already in the water surfing when Amelia, mum, and I arrived. Joshy and Ash came out of the water to wait for me, so I put on a wetsuit and we went out into the surf.

Not long after entering the surf, Karl joined us and took me out with him. Initially, we tried a few whitewashes to see how I handled it because obviously my body strength hadn't been tested in these conditions for many years. I hadn't been in the surf in a long time; it was interesting to see how my body held up.

I jumped onto the board and I paddled pretty easily to begin with. The further I went out against the waves, it started to get harder for me to paddle. Carl stood behind me and pushed my surfboard directly into the wave for me to catch it. This was my first attempt and I tried to stand up. It was crazy because my left leg came out from underneath me and naturally positioned itself as though I hadn't been away from the surf at all. For a few seconds, I actually stood on the board almost upright; Milz filmed it—I was so excited.

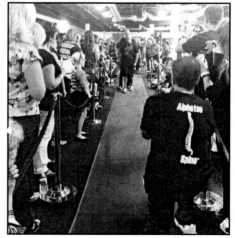

It had been probably 13 years since I last surfed, which was in Bali a few months before my accident. Yet here I was, attempting to get another piece of my life back, all these years later. I was still working through my recovery from the accident and it was like I hadn't been away from surfing at all. I struggled a little bit in the water—no excuses there—but it was so great to be out there and to get hit by a few waves. It was so amazing just to feel a bit weightless in the water!

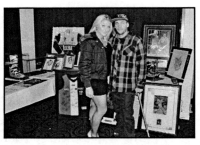

I only surfed with Joshy and the boys once during my time in Carlsbad. The number of training sessions I attended at Project Walk was enough to show my further improvement in my recovery. That surfing day with the boys was at the end of our trip and the weather was becoming colder there anyway. The boys had their scheduled races around the country to get on with, so they didn't get the chance to come back either, but at least I had the opportunity to do something that I previously enjoyed doing before my accident.

It was just another piece of my life that I got back. I had achieved another goal and it felt awesome.

I actually achieved three goals during that trip:
- To get back into the water and go surfing.
- To be able to actually stand up on the board (this was an extra bonus).
- To be able to get back to Project Walk and train hard enough so I could ditch my walking stick.

I used that stick for about nine years. It's amazing how quickly those years flew by. I just needed that challenge!

I think the moment that reality hit me was when I realized just how much I used my stick without consciously thinking about it. It was when we were walking back home from Project Walk one afternoon and Amelia asked me a question.

She looked straight at me and asked, "Why do you still use that stick?"

I said, "What do you mean?"

And Amelia said, "It's like a security blanket for you and you probably don't even really need it."

Her words really hit me. We had been at Project Walk for about eight weeks. My training was totally focused on getting myself to a recovery level where I could stand up, walk, sit down, and do whatever I wanted without having to use the stick.

What Amelia said was so simple and she said it in such a matter-of-fact manner. I did all this training but I still used the stick even when I was at the level of not needing to use it! The stick had become just what Amelia described it as: "a security blanket."

I thought it sounded a bit harsh, but it was definitely what I needed to hear.

So I asked myself the same question, "Why the hell am I still relying on this stick?"

It was like putting on a pair of shoes. I would get up to walk, and without a second thought, I would grab my stick and start walking off with it in my hand. It became a part of me. There was something within me that accepted that this walking stick was part of my life.

At Project Walk, I always concentrated on how I could get off it. I did all these exercises to strengthen my legs and get my balance back, and when I walked, I didn't need my stick. Sometimes I would walk normally and then my brain would take over—it would stuff me up and I would start walking in my own style again.

As I have said before, it's like getting an able-bodied person to walk like me. If they try to walk like me, then straight away their brain will go, "No, that's not right," and they will revert back to walking normally again.

My brain became so used to me walking in my style that it accepted it as normal for me, even though mentally I knew it was wrong and it looked wrong. I struggled to figure out what exactly the block was in my mentality that stopped me from correcting my walk. The thing only I knew was that whatever was blocking me was really deeply entrenched in my physical movement.

While we were in America, a friend of mine, who went through some traumatic injuries of his own and loved the alternative healing aspects, told me about a man who practiced a special type of hypnotherapy, which allowed the subconscious to go very deep—way past the patient's comfort levels. When he told me about his own experience, his only concern for me was that it could be very confronting, because it had the potential to bring me to the root of deep-seated issues that I might have locked away.

It sounded very intense, but after having so many mental blocks with my recovery on this trip, I decided to go and meet him to see what it was all about. Obviously my subconscious became used to the way I was and accepted that this style of walking was normal for me, even though I knew it wasn't.

A few days later, we caught up with the hypnotherapist; his name was Micco. We had a very in-depth chat about the type of healing technique he did, which was a form of deep Hypnotherapy based on American Native Indian Shaman healing principles. He said he might be able to help me break down a few barriers that I had stuck in my brain. I was on such a mission of not wanting to leave any stone unturned, but at the same time, I didn't want to take any risks mentally with the mindset part of my recovery.

I didn't know what negative thoughts I might have pushed to the back of my mind that I hadn't dealt with. I had worked very hard to get past all the unsupportive and "no hope" words that were drilled into me daily from the hospital and rehab teams. I needed to keep a clear and focused mindset on what I believed I could get back. I didn't want to undo any progress that I had made by bringing up negative emotions or feelings, but there was always a part of me that wanted to make sure that I didn't leave anything undone.

It took me a while to warm up to the idea of doing deep hypnosis, but the next time I saw him, I said, "Okay, lets try this."

I felt like I could trust this man to break though the negative beliefs I had buried deep inside my mind.

Amelia and I went to his place. He sat down with us and spent the first hour by doing a body map with me. We talked a lot about my injury. He told me about my physical structure and we went through my birthdate, astrology chart, and all that sort of information. It was actually very interesting. After a while, I felt comfortable enough with him and trusted him to guide me through his style of hypnotherapy.

He began by putting on some drumming music as background sound and he burned a special blend of herbs like incense. I smelled it straight away. It made me feel very relaxed and a bit sleepy.

I asked him, "What can I expect to get from this hypnotherapy session?"

He said that everybody's journey is different so he couldn't really tell me what I was going to see or connect to, or what would happen. He didn't even know what was going to happen on my own personal journey, but he assured me that I would be safe with him guiding me through the process.

He thought it might be easier if we did the process in shorter time-frames of just 15 minutes. So the first time, he got me focused on my breathing. I could really smell the incense he was burning and it went in through my mouth and nostrils, and right down into my lungs. I felt like I was smoking it.

I started to feel like I was losing control over everything. It felt like I was tumbling about in a washing machine. I didn't like it one bit! I couldn't control my thoughts; I couldn't control anything. I just kept fighting it the whole 15 minutes.

I came out of the session saying, "Nah, I don't like it. I don't like it at all."

I felt like I didn't achieve anything and I told him that. He said I had to stop fighting it. I had to relax and allow myself to go deep inside and go on my own journey.

The reality was that my legs just weren't working properly. As much as I did all the physical training, massaging, and things like that, I understood that I had deep-seated issues that I wasn't able to let go of, and now I had the best opportunity to break through them, by working with this shaman.

Because of my relentless search for answers and my "never give up" and "leave no stone unturned" attitude towards everything in life, I decided to give it another go.

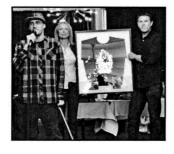

The second time I went into the hypnotic trance state, I tried to relax a lot more. I felt a total connection with my body. It was like the shell was removed and my body was resisting this removal at first, but then allowed me to go deep inside myself to a level I had never experienced before. It was like I connected to the part of my brain that controlled my dreams. When people dream, their pituitary gland becomes really active. I obviously connected in a big way, because the visions I had just went, *boom!* And I could clearly see all the nerves in my body, and I could identify every single nerve that no longer worked.

During this second time, the hypnotherapy technique had me in touch with my body so much that I could feel which nerves weren't contacting with different parts of my body.

Straight away I thought of Project Walk, when I did my walking training and how I would walk perfectly sometimes, but then my body would go, "No, this is not how you walk," and I would go back to the other style of walking that my body had grown accustomed to, which was unbalanced and awkward. That was the point I knew that it was going to be more of a mental game than a physical one.

I always knew there were so many things that I was able to do with my legs and that there was no physical reason why I couldn't do those things everyday. I had no other answers until I met Micco. I thought that since I hadn't tried this kind of healing before, I had nothing to lose and possibly everything to gain by trying it.

Determined to let everything go, I went in for the third and final session. This time, I actually went in deep right from the minute I closed my eyes, straight past all the bullshit conflicting thoughts and went, boom! I felt my body shake as if I was convulsing. It felt like my body was trying to shake out so much stuff: all the tension that I held onto, the restriction that kept me from moving freely, and all the spasms that contracted my muscles.

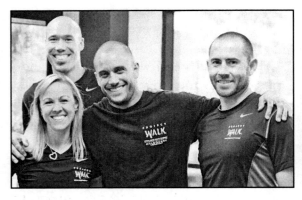

I knew I was rolling around on the ground but I couldn't stop. It all felt like a dream. I vaguely remember curling into a ball, and then I realized I had gone back to the time when I was a baby and still inside mum's womb. I looked to my left and I was able to see daylight through her skin. It was like looking through a thin red veil from the inside. I could feel my right arm and leg were jammed against the back of her, but my left side was free and relaxed, and then I started to come out of the hypnosis.

What I thought was interesting about that memory was that it was my right side that was affected in that moment in the womb. That was the same side of my body in exactly the same jammed-in, constricted position I experienced in my accident! I realized right then that I had two life events, but they were same life experience, even though they were many years apart.

It got me thinking that maybe part of my recovery needed me to go right back in time to before I was born in order to really understand the next level of my recovery.

While I witnessed that time of me being in mum's womb during the hypnosis session, I even made baby noises at one stage, like, *bebebebe*. It was weird because in my conscious mind I thought, *What the hell am I doing?*

But I couldn't stop making that noise. I could feel the vibrations in my body. I was having flashbacks of my life; I saw animals and spirit guides who guided me through this massive life journey, which is impossible to really explain to anyone else unless they have also experienced it. I saw a whole different world to what I normally see. I understood just how much my mind shut off, and how much potential I had to connect with my body and heal myself. It changed my whole perception of myself. Most importantly, this experience gave me the confidence to be able to get my body working the way it used to work before my accident.

Altogether, I had spent only a couple of hours with Micco. I felt like I did about 24 hours with him. I got so much out of the session, but I was totally exhausted and needed to go home and just chill.

When we got home, mum was there and I started to tell her about some of the things I saw while I was hypnotized:
- How I saw myself in her womb.
- How I saw my own birth.
- When I saw the way I was positioned in her womb with my right arm and my right leg stuck up against her back.

When I came out of the hypnosis session, I physically felt like my arm and leg were withered up. I told her how I was able to see through her skin and see daylight.

Mum explained my birth. I was a forceps delivery and I was premature by two weeks. The weird thing was that I knew I was a forceps delivery, but I hadn't been told by mum or anyone else that I was two weeks premature before she told me just then.

Amelia told me that during one of the sessions, I kept saying, "I'm not ready, I'm not ready."

I explained my whole birth to mum in detail of what it was like for me.

Mum just said, "What you have just described to me is exactly how you were born."

Mum couldn't believe the experience I had with Micco and the detailed information about my birth that I was able to get through the hypnosis session.

She said to me, "Wow, this is huge!"

I thought it was amazing how far I went back in my life journey—right to being a baby in mum's womb.

Later after Amelia got her mind around what she witnessed as I went through the hypnotherapy session, she said it was like watching an exorcism at times. She said she watched me go through my accident all over again.

When I had my accident, I obviously suppressed a lot of emotion by trying to keep calm and not panic. When I was under hypnosis, all of that suppressed pain and fear came out.

Amelia said that I kept saying, "You're not taking me, I'm not ready to go, I'm not ready to go!"

It was as if I was yelling at someone who was trying to take me somewhere else. I felt so terrible for Amelia because I didn't know it was going to play out like that. I had hypnotherapy sessions before and I looked like I was asleep, but this was a whole new level of hypnotherapy.

I understood that I had suppressed so much—especially since the accident. I hadn't released the pain properly. I realized that I had 12 years of accident pain to release and it all blazed out in that hypnotherapy session.

I felt more at peace afterwards, but only after about a week or two later when I had more time to process all the information that came up. I had such a different outlook on the world. I didn't have a fear of my accident anymore. I didn't have a fear of letting go of my walking stick and relying just on my two legs, or relying upon Amelia if I happened to stumble. Whether that was a result of the work I did with Micco, or with Project Walk, or with Uschi, I walked into Project Walk and ditched my walking stick! I symbolically broke it in half. I knew I didn't need it anymore. Over the years, I tried at least 20 times to ditch that walking stick, but I would start to use it again a couple of hours later.

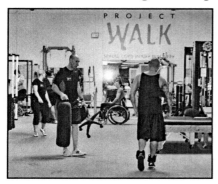

I think the combination of those three elements—Uschi, Micco, and Project Walk—unlocked a lot of deep-seated things and opened up my mind to so many possibilities. The work I did with Micco showed me a lot of things I didn't want to see, but I learned how I could resolve them and move forward from them. Uschi worked on the spiritual side of me; she was able to unlock stuff on that level and clear a lot of negativity out—especially the fear I was holding onto about my seizure.

With everything I worked with and with everyone who worked on me, I gained my physical and inner strength back. I had this power and strength in me. I had lost it for a while there, but now I had this fire in me again.

I continued to get my recovery from alternative practices and therapies. I achieved my greatest results from them without a doubt.

It has always been my belief that if I did everything possible and gave everything a go, then at least I could say that I gave it 100 percent and left no stone unturned. I applied that belief to every aspect of my life, especially to my recovery.

I have learned that it is important to be well informed and to educate myself about recovery and healing, and to do my research on all the different therapies and techniques available to me. As long as there's proof that other people have gone through it, achieved results from it, and are happy and 100 percent satisfied with the recovery path they chose, then I think there is no harm in trying it, whether it's conventional or unconventional.

As I have said before, everyone is different. It doesn't always work the same way for everybody, but I'm a big believer in trying anything, and that's why I looked at everything that was available to me. From all the information and evidence I had, I chose to go with the alternative healing path to get my results and help my recovery.

This was just another part of my life that I needed to do and I don't regret it. It was amazing how much I grew as a person during these alternative therapies. I don't even think about grabbing my walking stick anymore when I get up from having lunch, or get up from sitting down for long periods of time, or even when I'm going out.

But there is always the flip side to it.

It's really hard sometimes, and I don't walk as far as I used to. It's way more stress on my body and on my brain because I'm thinking about so much more stuff, such as the distance I have to walk, the surface I have to walk on, the obstacles I need to manoeuvre around, or the people I have to be mindful not to bump into or have them crash into me. Even with all this stuff I have to figure out as I'm walking along, for me, the walking stick was about just letting go of something that was holding me back rather than something I used that helped me walk.

I'm sure that with time, I will start to move easier and get better at walking by myself. I'll get a lot stronger so I'll be able to walk further distances without having to stop, but right now, I have to go through this stage.

It was exactly the same as when I got out of the wheelchair. One day I decided that I didn't need the wheelchair anymore, and instantly my mobility and the distance I was able to cover became a lot more challenging. I couldn't go as far as I used to and I couldn't get around as quickly. I had all those same difficulties, but I made that decision to finally get out of the wheelchair because I didn't want to have that as part of me. It was like a massive layer came off me, and the walking stick was another layer that came off me. I didn't realize how much I relied on that walking stick.

For many years I didn't even think to get off it because it is much more difficult to ditch the stick, because of all the reasons I mentioned above. But, it is another layer that I have to let go of and I'm grateful for that; I'm getting so much better not using it.

It has been 13 years since my accident, and I have to at least acknowledge how far I have come and what I have achieved. I have transitioned through many stages to get to where I am today—to be able to walk unaided. From the beginning of the wheelchair, to the elbow crutches, the foot orthotic, the walking stick, and now—to no aid at all.

My recovery journey was a long and arduous one, so when I broke the walking stick, it was more than just snapping an old stick. I broke off all my reliance on anything that helped me walk!

This was my next stage of life—walking one foot in front of the other one step at a time. And it was awesome!

# Chapter 8

# When Life Gives You Lemons, Squeeze With All You've Got!

## From sweet to sour and back to sweet times again.

A few months after I got out of rehab in 2001, I spent some time down at Dingo's mum's house. He was back from America for a month or two, so the boys and myself went to chill at his place, go to house parties, and just be boys. His mum's place was on a large plot of land, so we brought my dirt bike down so I could ride it around the property. I had only bought it a few months before my accident so I didn't really have a chance to enjoy it. As I looked at my bike right there in front of me, I couldn't wait to get on it. I stood out of my chair and the boys lifted me onto it. It felt so great to sit back on my bike. Hearing my bike start up, and smelling the fuel and oil bought up so many exciting memories.

I had decent movement in my left leg, so I could use the gears. I pulled in the clutch, kicked it into first gear, and took off! Apart from my lack of core strength, it was just awesome! I felt really confident being back on the bike and riding around.

I clicked second. Obviously I had to do some small wheelies to impress the boys! It took a lot of convincing to get me to stop, but when I did, the feeling of freedom was so overwhelming—almost to the point that it brought me happy tears. This feeling of freedom gave me so much more drive to keep going with my fitness.

Not long after I returned home to Melbourne from America from my time with Dana and John, mum went over there with my Grandma. They met up with a distant relative in San Francisco who was a cousin of mum's, and they hit it off really quick. He owned a winery in Northern California and to cut a long story short, he offered mum an opportunity to be part of his wine business. Mum was to export premium quality wines from Australia under his American label, but before this could happen, she had to go to America and learn about his winery and his existing range of wines. This was a great offer for mum as she already had contacts in the Australian boutique wine industry.

When she came home and told me about this, I was so excited for her. I encouraged her to do it. We talked a lot about it; it was a huge decision for us both. Finally we felt it was an opportunity to start new lives with new people in a new country. So a few months later, mum moved to Sonoma in California. Her first day at the winery was 11 September 2001. I joined mum there a month later. I was originally meant to go earlier but since it was when the attacks on New York happened, I waited in Australia an extra few weeks before joining her.

It was great being in Sonoma. Mum was happy in her new role and I got along with my new distant cousin and his daughter really well. It also gave me the chance to start my new life with people who didn't know the old Josh, so there wasn't any sadness around me.

We lived in mum's cousin's home. I trained in his home gym every day, rode my push-bike, which I had learned to ride again, around the beautiful Sonoma streets. My riding wasn't always pretty but I managed, and things were going well. I really enjoyed life at the winery. Some weekends, I helped out as the concierge by welcoming guests and spotting the big buyers, which I was really good at. I also developed a taste for Sauvignon Blanc and Pinot Noir. I still enjoy my cousin's Sauvignon Blanc to this day and still enjoy a great Pinot!

Life in America was going well, but I had to return to Australia to organize a few things: sell my car, see my dad for his birthday, and spend Christmas with mum's family and as well as with my dad's family. When I got home, it felt great to be there. I loved being in America, but I only had a few friends there and I was limited as to what I could do—I was only 19 years old.

Within that month, I made the tough choice to stay in Australia. Things were good at home. I had my mates and freedom to do what I wanted, which is exactly what I did.

Without mum to keep me focused, I realized that I had become a little self-destructive. I wasn't training as much; I was more focused on catching up on the things I had missed for the past 18 months. I didn't live with my aunt anymore because she had had enough of me. I can see why, and I don't blame her—I was pretty out of control! I found it really hard to stick to her rules and routines. I lived between different friends' houses over a two-month period, and in that time, I met a girl and I decided I definitely wasn't going back to America then.

When I told mum that I had decided to stay in Melbourne, she didn't take it too well. She loved being there, even though she was having a tough time financially. But, I was sure I didn't want to go back. In February 2002, mum decided to come home to Melbourne. I was a little out of control and mum was struggling a bit in America, so she moved back to Australia. We ended up renting a house in Port Melbourne. Mum got back into her old line of work, and I was happily in a relationship. I was back to riding motocross bikes at my girlfriend's family's property. I still trained a little bit, but not as much as I should have. I was too busy trying to be a kid and have fun.

My girlfriend and I were both young, and it soon became a very toxic relationship. It was very hard at times. In successful relationships, it is important to live in part for the other person; this was very frustrating for me because it always reminded of the things I couldn't do. These things included even the most simple activities that couples just do together and expect to be able to do together, like go for long walks or do adventurous things. I always tried, but sometimes I got the feeling it wasn't enough, and being young as we were, we just wanted to get the most out of life and share that with each other. As much as I wanted to be able to all those things with ease, it just didn't work that way for me.

A year later, as I moved through my recovery, it was important for me to get back into doing some of the things I did before my accident. I needed to reestablish in my mind and in my body the things that I did and I enjoyed doing.

I wasn't Josh the quadriplegic; I was Josh with the injury. My injury slowed me down from doing a lot of things in life, but I could still do them. Injuries should not stop anyone from doing anything altogether.

My ultimate goal was to get more and more of my old life back. I realized that I just had to keep working at it, just chip away, get fit, and believe!

I decided to introduce back into my life all those things that I loved to do. Just being on the snow was one of these things. I was determined to bring snowboarding back into my life—the one thing I was most passionate about! My new goal was to go back to the snow and try to snowboard again.

My girlfriend and I returned to the mountain where I had my accident—the same mountain that had changed the course of my life just three years before. Mum was coming up on the Sunday.

We met Chrisso and Daniel at the resort. It was so surreal to be back there. Other than the weekend in September 2000, when mum and I went up there so I could see the jump site and gave me some clarity with what had gone wrong with the jump, I hadn't been near the snow. So many thoughts and emotions were running through me, and I didn't know what to think or what to do! The best part was the snow was fresh, there was good cover, and the weather was clear but cold; so it was perfect for me to get back to what I loved. We spent the Saturday hanging out with friends; I decided not to board until Sunday. I was still very weak and I didn't want to push myself.

Above all that, I was beyond excited to be back in the snow. On Sunday the weather conditions on the mountain were just perfect for the day that I returned to boarding again. It was a beautiful sunny day; the snow was still really fresh, the visibility was great, and I could see forever into the distance!

Daniel's dad Geoff put me on a snowmobile and took me over to one of the runs. I was so nervous and excited at the same time. I had no clue how my legs were going to react but I was willing to give it another crack.

Daniel slid over to me, helped me strap into my board, and he said, "Alright bud, you ready?"

Hell yeah I was ready!

It was around 2 p.m. and fortunately the mountain was not very busy. With some help from Daniel and his dad, they lifted me to my feet. Daniel held onto my hands and we slowly started to slide down the hill. It was the best feeling; hearing the snow under my board, the wind in my face, and being back up on the snow for the first time in three years.

My boarding was sketchy to say the least. Daniel only just let go when I demanded to let me try by myself. My legs surprisingly held up better than I expected. I definitely didn't ride like I used to, but I didn't care—I was back on a board only three years after my accident! There we were—Daniel, Chrisso, and me—slowly boarding down the slope. I couldn't believe how much all my hard training had paid off!

Mum skied ahead and took photographs of us as we boarded down the run. She had happy tears while she skied next to me and watched me get back another piece of my life. Then towards the bottom of the run, mum went ahead to take some more photos of Daniel, Chrisso, and me. As we got closer to mum, Daniel let go of me so I was boarding without any help. I had my two best mates riding side-by-side next to me like the old days. Mum snapped pictures like crazy capturing us riding. She captured a great shot of us three riding down the hill. It was probably one of the best feelings I have ever had even to this day! That afternoon, for the first time in nearly three years, I had so much freedom with my boys at a place I loved most doing the very thing I loved most.

This moment was huge for me and definitely worth capturing on film. I was so determined to get back up there again, but since it was the end of the season, I would have to wait until next year. At least I knew that I had a future with boarding even if the jumping days were over.

## Kay

All along, our goal was for Josh to get his life back. Our lack of understanding of spinal cord injury allowed us to live in a sort of "ignorance is bliss" state as far as his recovery was concerned.

When Josh decided to go to the snow again, I was scared, but I knew that Josh hadn't gone through all he had to not at least try the things he loved doing before his accident. As his mum, I was always nervous that something would go wrong. He knew I could only handle one spinal cord injury, so if he did anything stupid and reinjured himself, he wouldn't have me in his corner. It sounds tough, but the mental trauma was something I couldn't deal with again. I knew that Josh knew this, so I trusted him to be careful and to evaluate any activity he was doing.

So the bookings were made for the snow trip. It was decided that he would relax on the mountain on the Saturday then board on the Sunday. I coped with so much flack from everybody for agreeing to this, but I simply said that Josh had earned the right to get on with his life, so I totally supported what he was doing.

I called Paula and asked her what she thought. She came back to me later and said it would be okay but Josh couldn't start snowboarding until 2 p.m. on Sunday. If he waited until then, it would be perfect! Josh had learned to respect Paula's views so he agreed to wait until 2 p.m.

I was positive, excited, and a little scared, but I knew I had to support Josh.

It was a beautiful sunny Sunday; I drove up to the mountain from Port Melbourne in my sports car. The weather was so amazing! I had the roof down for the whole trip, which took around three hours. When I arrived there, the mountain was beautiful. The sunshine was brilliant and the snow was perfect.

Although I had been a keen skier before Josh's accident, I hadn't skied since, so it was my first time back skiing in three years. I hired my gear and met Josh, his girlfriend, and the boys. We were all so excited.

Josh got up to the slopes as soon as it was 2 p.m. and he was off with the boys. I skied in front of them and took photos. I managed to get some great shots once Josh became more confident on his own with the boys boarding next to him.

It was a huge moment for us all. It was just one more thing that we could cross off the bucket list of Josh getting his life back. There were many happy tears!

My life really started to come back together and I felt the most positive about my future that I had felt in a long time. I looked forward to unfolding the next chapter.

One day, I received a letter that would determine the direction of one very important area of my life. Mum had taken out an accident insurance on herself not long before my accident. She decided to take out an accident policy on me as well. When I had my accident, the insurance company told us that I was eligible for a $470,000 payout! In those days, that amount of money would have set me up with a home and a reasonable amount to invest.

For over three years, our lawyers went back and forth with the insurance company about my accident claim. We finally got the letter we were waiting for from the insurance company. We were so excited as mum read it out, but then I watched her face change from a happy face and slowly drop to a sad face and into tears. Within seconds, she just broke down right in front of me.

I said, "Mum what's wrong? What has happened?"

She brought herself back together and read the letter out loud.

It stated, "We have studied Josh's injury and recovery. Since he walked in the first year it is apparent to us that Josh is not entitled to the full amount … We are willing to make an offer to Josh of a total payout of $1,300."

What was really frustrating was that even my latest MRIs showed there had been no improvement in my spinal cord. I was still presenting as a complete quadriplegic. The swelling in my spinal cord had gone, but it was still crushed. This just knocked the wind out of us!

For the last three years, mum had spent every cent she had to help my recovery. She even sold her art collection. She had built up a lot of debt since my accident by paying for my many recovery programs. She wasn't too worried because we always thought the insurance payout would allow her to get rid of the debt and that I would be able to buy a house. I felt like I had been punished for doing well with my injury. Against all odds and medical predictions, I had walked, yet the insurance company would not give us a rightful payout. This just broke our hearts, but we had no choice.

What we were definitely not going to take was the $1,300 payout offer. That wouldn't have even paid for the x-ray bills. There was no use staying upset about it, because the insurance company had made their decision and we all just had to get on with life as best we could. We just carried on like we always did. We picked ourselves up, reminded ourselves that there is someone worse off than us, and kept moving forward.

It was a stressful time and we all felt it on some level. The relationship with my girlfriend became harder and harder and I wasn't sure if we would stay together.

One day Dutchy came over with his new puppy Tilly. She was a little Staffy—what we call Staffordshire Bull Terriers. I just loved her when I met her. Mum loved Tilly too. We talked about getting a dog for me as a companion. We always had dogs in our lives in the past, so we decided the time was right for me to get a puppy. I was so excited because the last three years had been so tough in more ways than one, and getting a puppy gave me a new companion that I could look forward to having with me.

That night, we got the Trading Post newspaper and looked through the "Dogs for Sale" section. We found an advertisement for American Staffordshire pups, so I called them straight away and we arranged to go out there the next day to see them.

When we pulled up in the car, Mum said, "Okay, we're not going to get the first puppy we see."

I agreed with her, but that soon changed when we saw the mamma of the litter—she was beautiful. Next, all the puppies greeted us and I was given this little orange-red bundle of joy to hold. I just fell in love with her straight away, but I didn't want to rush into buying the first puppy I held. I looked at all of them.

There were so many that I didn't know which one to choose, so we put them all in the basket and I said, "Whichever one comes straight to me, I'll take."

As soon as they were let back out of the basket, the same pup I had originally held ran straight to me, stopped, turned around, and sat right down on my foot!

Mum and the breeders laughed and said, "Well I think you have been chosen."

I was so excited! We came back two days later and picked her up. We named her Montana. I just fell head over heels in love with her. Since then, it has been 10 years and she has never left my side.

Montana is my best friend.

A month passed since we got Montana, and having her in my life made me realize I needed to get out of the toxic relationship that I had with my girlfriend. One of my biggest fears with having my injury was that I would never find anyone who would want to be with me or who could deal with my recovery issues. So while I was in the relationship, even though it was getting really bad, I thought that she was the only girl who would want to be with me. Having that fear made me doubt myself, and because of that I put up with a lot of shit from her. I wasn't a perfect boyfriend, but I never lied or cheated. There was a lot of jealousy from both sides, and because we were both so young, it clearly showed. Once Montana came into my life and gave me unconditional love, I realized that I could still be just as happy on my own.

A month later, we both came to the understanding that our relationship was going nowhere and we parted ways. Having Montana in my life kept me focused. She gave me a purpose and a responsibility to keep healthy, strong, and active.

I was just over three years post-accident. One thing that I noticed was that my recovery went through continuous highs and lows. There was no consistency to my recovery. There were I was never times when I was just completely well all of the time. I was going through a low period where my recovery started to slow down and I had dark thoughts and demons that haunted me at night.

Somehow, Montana could sense my upset feelings and she always comforted me. It was as though she just *knew*, and I'm sure that if it weren't for her, then I would have gone through depression after three years of all the unsettling ups and downs I had experienced in my life. Montana made such a huge difference in my life. She was my best friend and she went everywhere with me. There wasn't a minute in my day that she wasn't by my side.

Fortunately, not all insurance companies were as brutal as the first one was to me in regards to my recovery. Just over three years after my accident, I received a payment through my superannuation insurance. It was paid because, in their eyes and assessment, I was "Totally Permanently Disabled" through my accident. Mum and I talked about it, and we decided that I should buy myself my dream car as a reward for all my hard work: a green General Motors Holden "SS" utility vehicle with black leather seats.

Montana would sit on the leather passenger seat in my Ute next to me and look out the window. Her favourite spot was lying on the seat with her head on my lap

My mates would say to me, "Josh, why don't you cover the seats with a sheet to protect the leather from Montana?"

And I would reply, "I don't put a sheet down when you get in the car so why would I for Montana? Who cares if the seats get scratched? As long as she's next to me and happy, I don't care!"

Monny was my little buddy, my saviour; she filled my void when my mind went to dark places.

Over the next two years not very much changed. I kept up with my full-time job of recovering and getting better.

During that time, I visited people with spinal cord injuries in rehab and in the same hospital as I was admitted to when I had my accident. Either the patients or their families contacted me after hearing about my story and recovery. I never gave advice and I never made promises. I just simply told my story. I always made sure that they understood that every spinal cord injury is different.

I made a few visits and saw different people. I chatted with them and their family support teams, asked them about their injury and how they were doing with theirs, and shared my own story about my injury and recovery.

On one of my last visits to rehab, some of the people with spinal cord injuries and their family members spoke to me quietly and informed me that the staff at the rehab and hospital asked these families what I was doing coming back in there.

When the families and the person with the injury told the staff the reason for my visits, the staff told the injured person and their family support team to not listen to me since I gave people "false hope" and I "was never as bad as I said I was."

I became tired of hearing this, so I decided to get new MRIs of my injury and send them to a surgeon in Sydney who knew absolutely nothing about my recovery or outcome of my cord injury. He was recommended to us through a friend of mum's. He was very highly regarded. A few weeks later, mum and I flew up to Sydney to meet with him. As I walked into his room, he looked at me with this startled expression on his face and directed his gaze past me as if someone was standing behind me.

As I sat down, he said to me, "You can't be Josh Wood!"

I replied, "Of course I am. I just flew up from Melbourne to meet you."

He replied, "That's impossible! I was expecting you to be in a chair!"

I laughed and said, "Tell me something I haven't heard! Yes, I'm Josh Wood and yes, those MRIs on your desk are 100 percent mine."

He then sat down and said, "Josh, I am so astounded in your recovery. In my years of practice I have never seen a recovery like yours."

He then went on to explain that my cord damage was still very apparent. He also explained that my cord had deteriorated so much that it shrunk to a minimal amount with only 5 percent working function. He clipped my MRI film onto the light box and flicked on the light switch.

I freaked out! It scared the shit out of me to see my injury so highlighted. I immediately became very upset.

I thought, *Anytime now it could snap and I will get worse.*

I had come all this way in my recovery and now I had this hanging over my head. He saw that I was quite distressed after seeing the image of my injury on the light box and from hearing his opinion.

After having more of a positive chat with the doctor and mum, they convinced me that it was a remarkable recovery I had achieved. The doctor felt it wouldn't get any worse.

I was worried that if I got a knock to the neck it would snap the cord, the doctor told me, "Josh, someone could hit you over the back of the neck with a baseball bat and it wouldn't make a difference. Your neck has been fused. The bat would most likely break before your neck or the cord would."

I laughed and said, "That would be a good party trick!"

He said, "You definitely shouldn't try it, but don't worry about it. You've been living with it for many years like this, so don't let any of these thoughts stop you from doing anything else."

It was so nice to meet a positive surgeon who had a great attitude towards my recovery. He also wrote a summary with his prognosis, which we still have to this date, and it is proof that I was actually that bad and I still am!

Mum and I were glad that we travelled up to Sydney to meet with that surgeon. We now had the undeniable evidence, which stated the extent of my injury and proved to anyone who didn't believe that my injury was as bad as I claimed it to be. I wasn't trying to prove anything, but when I go to see someone with a spinal cord injury, I want them to know that I am the real deal and I know what I am talking about!

## Kay

My business was going well, so I decided to look for a small ground floor two-bedroom apartment nearby so that Josh could move into it to make things easier for him.

I was taking Montana for a walk, and I met my sister in front of the Old Church redevelopment in town Port Melbourne. There was a small "For Sale" sign on the gate.

I said to Wendy, "I should look at this."

So, we rang the agent, and arranged for an inspection later that morning. I didn't say anything to Josh. Wendy and I went through it and it was perfect. Not just for Josh, but for me and Montana also. I was too scared to ask what the price was. The agent said it had been sold twice, but had fallen through on finance.

She said, "Make an offer!"

Wendy and I sat down. I called Josh and he came around straight away. The minute he walked in, he loved the place.

And I said, "Well I am going to make an offer."

He said, "Mum, don't do this to me. I just love it—we have to get it."

I worked quickly through what I had in savings, figured out what I would get for my old apartment, and made an offer. Within 24 hours, they accepted it. It was a fair offer, but nowhere near what it was worth. We found out later that there were two other offers that weekend, which were much higher than mine, but ours was the one accepted. So it was ours; we had a new place to live.

I really believed that the universe ensured I got that apartment.

After our visit with the surgeon in Sydney, we went back home to Melbourne and I went straight back into my training routine. Rather than go to the gym and be indoors every time I trained, I did some less strenuous exercises in mum's backyard. We had moved house two more times in those two years, and then finally settled into our dream home in Port Melbourne. It was a ground floor apartment in a renovated church. When mum bought it, it had two bedrooms, one bathroom, and a huge living room, which could have fitted two full-sized pool tables. It was originally designed to be commercial offices.

Mum decided to build my own area in the apartment, so we ripped the carpet up and drew the plan on the concrete slab. Mum's cousin's husband Paul, a builder, turned the large open area into a bedroom with an en suite bathroom and separate living room just for me, and it also included a private rear courtyard, so I basically had my own one-bedroom apartment. The whole renovation was done around me while I was living there. It was a mess, but it ended up being a really great space.

The apartment had a large yard with two big palm trees. It was on the corner of one of Port Melbourne's busiest cross streets. The boys and myself called our yard "The Beer Garden."

It was such an awesome backyard. We spent hours in it having BBQs, beers, and laughs. Every weekend in the summer it was party central.

That year, Chrisso lived with us for a nearly four months when he was in between jobs, which was a lot of fun.

Chrisso was a groomer up on the mountain, so he cleaned up all the runs in a Kässbohrers; he built jumps and created the snow park.

When the snow season started the year after I resumed snowboarding, and Chrisso had moved back up to the snow; he convinced me to come up and stay for one weekend. Well, that one weekend end turned into six weeks! I moved into Chrisso's apartment with him and two others. I spent a few days up there then a few days back in Melbourne with mum and Montana. Up on the mountain I went out on the slopes and snowboarded—well, I tried to—and it got frustrating at times but I always reminded myself that I was lucky to be able to do it on my own.

Most of my time there was spent at the local pub with Chrisso and our other friends. It was a great six weeks and one night I went night boarding and rode exactly how I used to ride except for the jumps. The conditions were perfect and it all clicked for me that one night. The next day I went back to struggling on the board, so after that I decided to let the snowboarding go and just remember it how it used to be and move on. I was missed Montana a lot and I was getting tired of the constant partying. I needed structure back in my life.

It was near the end of the season, so I went back to mum's apartment, got back into a good routine, and enjoyed being back home away from the crazy lifestyle up on the mountain.

I met a girl and we started a relationship. This one quickly became toxic and showed up all the classic mistakes. History was just repeating itself.

I had learned from my last relationship that I shouldn't stay in a toxic environment, so after about 10 months, we parted ways. The one great thing to come out of this relationship was that she introduced me to two brothers who were her friends at the time; their names were Boz and Alex. We clicked straight away and we became instant best mates. When my girlfriend and I broke up, the boys still stayed in my life because we had an awesome friendship. They pretty much lived at our place. They came over most nights after work and we went out riding dirtbikes on the weekends and hit up the strip clubs on the usual Friday and Saturday nights. We used to go to nightclubs, but there were always hassles with crowds and "heroes" giving me a hard time over my walk. We needed somewhere to hang out and we discovered strip clubs. They weren't as crowded, security was always good, and the girls mostly became our friends.

Boz and Alex were great mates! They were always there for me when I needed them and they were fun to hang with.

Not long after meeting Boz and Alex, my friend Lukey Luke introduced me to young kid named Zayne. I met him one day when we were watching Lukey ride. Straight away I took Zayne under my wing. He was like a little brother to me. Like Boz and Alex, Zayne was at our place a few times a week. He would come to the strip clubs with us but the difference was that Zayne was only sixteen. That never bothered us; the clubs security never questioned him because he had the look and attitude of someone much older than his years. The looks on the faces of the club's security guys were hilarious, when two years later, we were celebrating Zayne's birthday at the same strip club we went to every week.

When security asked how old he turned, they were a little shocked when I said, "Agh it's his eighteenth."

Montana loved having all the boys over, mum definitely got over it at times but they were always respectful and never damaged anything. If something broke, then they always replaced it.

One day not long after meeting Zayne, mum was patting Montana.

She suddenly stopped and said to me, "Josh, what's this?"

I went over and felt a big hard lump in Montana's neck near her throat. The next day I took her to our vet. The news broke my heart. It was cancer. They had to perform surgery straight away.

I was destroyed as I left the vet's practice without her because I didn't know if she was going to be okay. The look on Montana's face tore me apart. One minute she was in full puppy mode running amuck, but then I handed the lead to the vet and kissed her goodbye and walked off.

She quickly stopped panting, sat down, and tilted her head to the side, as if to say, "Dad, wait, where are you going? What about me?"

I didn't stop crying until later the next day when the vet called me and said, "Josh, great news, we were able to get all the cancer! It was only in one spot and she can come home later today."

It felt like a huge weight had been lifted off my shoulders! The boys and mum where equally as excited about the news, but mum was worried. She saw how destroyed I was when I didn't know if I was going to lose Montana. She said that maybe I should think about getting another dog in case something happened to her. Another dog would not replace Montana in any way, but it was more about sharing the love between two furry buddies instead of one. At the time, I wasn't having it.

I said, "No way! No dog would replace Montana!"

I loved having just her. I loved her so much and she was totally spoilt. I didn't think it would be fair on another dog, and especially not fair on Montana. I didn't want the focus to be taken off her and risk changing the big personality that she already had.

A few months later, my mates Blacky and Kazza's dog, had a litter of American bulldog pups. They randomly sent me a picture of them, to see if I knew anyone that might want to buy one. I just fell in love with these cute little pups, and thought that maybe it would be a good idea for Monny to have a little friend. A week later mum and I went down to check them out; mum fell in love with them until she met their dad, big Al. He came bouncing over with a truck tire in his mouth!

Mum freaked and said, "Josh, no way! They are huge. You cannot have one of them in an apartment."

I was gutted, but couldn't fight her on that one. I told Zayne about the awesome little pup I had been thinking of getting, and said, maybe he might want him. That weekend Zayne went down and bought the same pup.

A few weeks later, Paula came over to visit us. She said she would give me a reading. In the middle of the reading, she started going on about this little bundle of joy waiting for me. She started to describe a tiny white puppy and I immediately knew what she was talking about.

I said, "Oh yeah, Blacky's puppies! You must be talking about the puppy I was going to get, but Zayne got him."

Straight away she said, "No, there's another in the same litter but a different pup. You didn't notice him but he noticed you when you visited a few weeks ago. Thor's waiting for you."

I said, "How did you know I wanted to name the original pup Thor?" She just looked at me and laughed.

She said, "Your mum won't be happy, but she will realize very quickly that he is a very special puppy."

Without hesitation, I called mum and told her what Paula just told me. Mum agreed that if there was a male pup left, then we would trial him for two weeks. I called Blacky straight away and asked if there were any males left.

He said, "Yeah there's one left, Thor's waiting for you."

And I freaked out! Blacky knew I wanted to name the original pup Thor, but when he said that he was waiting for me, I knew it was him! The next day, Boz, Alex, and I went to Kazza's and Blacky's house and picked up Thor. There he was—all dirty from playing in the yard. He ran straight to me and jumped into my arms. We had to wash him three times before we got him white again and clean enough that we could bring him home. I put him in the backyard. I wanted to let Montana find him, and she did! Montana loved Thor straight away, until she realized that he wasn't leaving. It took her about a week to warm up to him, but after that, we never had a worry. She used to treat him like a toy. She would grab onto his wrinkly face and drag him around the yard in a playful manner, and he would just let her. He just stayed floppy and allowed himself to be dragged along; they were best mates.

One night, when Zayne, Boz, Alex, Ross, and I were out, I was introduced to this guy Laslo. Laslo used to race motocross so we had a few common friends. After that first night of meeting Laslo, I knew I had met someone who would be my best mate for the rest of my life.

Laslo and I hung out nearly every single day; we rode dirtbikes on the weekdays and weekends, partied hard, and went on road trips all the time. We hit the beaches with our dogs; Laslo always had his two dogs in the back of his Ute. At that time, I had a big American truck: an F250. I would put my dogs in the back of my truck and we would take them to the motor cross tracks and on road trips. We had such a fun summer; all of us—Laslo, Boz, Alex, Zayne, the dogs, and the rest of our mates.

We went up to visit a holiday home up on the Murray River, which belonged to another mate of mine, Mitch. We went out on his family's speedboat all day along the river, and then at night we had fun at the clubs and pubs. We had such a good time. There was never any drama because we always had each other's backs.

It was about seven or eight years post-accident and I was really getting on with my life. I was still using the walking stick, but I hadn't been in my wheelchair for about six years.

Not long after meeting Laslo, I met a girl and got into another relationship. If I thought that my last two relationships were toxic, then I was in for a big surprise! She was also pretty young, so I guess I had coming. I should have listened to mum and the boys, but I had to follow my already predictable pattern and learn the hard way! We didn't last long, and once it was over—again—I went back to focusing upon what meant the world to me—my boys, my dogs, and my freedom. By this point, I had had three strikes—or relationships—and I was out. I can honestly say that my relationships with those "girlfriends" gave me more grief than my injury!

## Kay

The five years or so that we lived in the old church were happy times for us all. It was a time of healing for us both and the dogs were very happy there too. Eventually, the upkeep of the garden and the constant partying got to me. As much as I loved the boys, I needed some space, and I knew that Josh needed to get his own place to commence his life away from me, so we decided to sell it in 2009. While it was sad, it was just a necessary part of us both getting on with our own lives. My promise to Josh all those years ago was to help him get his independence back so this was the next chapter.

In 2009, mum decided to sell our apartment. We had spent about five years there and we had so many fun memories of living in the old church. I guess it was time for mum to get her own life back and get away from my entourage and me, and we really couldn't blame her for that. Mum bought herself a smaller apartment in Port Melbourne, and I bought a big home in the outer western suburbs of Melbourne, right near Laslo's new home, which was also close to Boz and Alex's house. Zayne decided that it was time for him to move out of his parents' house, so he came live with me.

Zayne and I had a huge house all to ourselves, so about two or three months later, another mate of ours named Jadeo moved into the house with us. Now we had even more fun!

There wasn't a day when we didn't have all the other boys over; I loved every minute of it. I finally had more independence and had my mates with me 24/7. I ended up selling my F250 truck to buy another vehicle: a brand new red General Motors Holden SS Ute. I had sold my truck for more than I bought it for so I was able to get the new car. I was in love with my new bright red Ute; Laslo had one too so we had twin cars. The neighbors must have thought something suspicious was going on in that house. Most of my mates had brand new cars and we lived in the biggest house on the block. Every weekend, we had big BBQs and roast lamb-on-the-spit feasts. It was one of my best summer experiences ever.

One weekend, a good friend of mine, Gav Walker, called me up. He owns a Harley Davidson motorcycle dealership in a big country town called Mildura in Northern Victoria. Gav and I had been speaking about getting me back on a Harley, and he told me that my good mate Maddo (Robbie Maddison) was arriving that coming weekend. Gav said that I should fly up for a boy's weekend. Robbie was testing a long distance jump at Gav's, so I jumped at the opportunity to fly up and see them both. Little did I know what Gav and Maddo had planned for me! I booked my ticket the minute I got off the phone, and I flew up a few days later.

Gav's daughter Annie and his wife Kazza—a different Kazza—picked me up from the airport and took me straight to meet Gav and his son Jack, who were already at the jump site prepping it for Maddo's arrival.

Soon after getting there, Gav, Jack, and I went back to "Quick-Fix," which was Gav's Harley shop.

Gav said to me, "Alright Wood boy, which Harley do you want to ride? We gotta go meet Maddo about 100 kilometers' out of town, and we're going now so be quick."

I had no time to be nervous even though it was my first time on a Harley since my accident. I chose a bike and we were off. It was just like my dream I had 10 years prior, back when I was in ICU—the one of me riding a Harley with my mates, feeling free and knowing I had my life back—it was so surreal! Gav said he could see the smile on my face in his mirror throughout the entire ride.

We met Maddo on the side of the road. He didn't know I was coming up with Gav, and he really surprised to see me on a Harley, which set the tone for the next few days. They couldn't get me off the Harley nor did they try!

The first day, Maddo jumped all day, and at lunch, Gav took us to the local pub and ordered 60 Oysters Kilpatrick for only four of us. After watching Maddo jump, I felt the itch to try it myself, but obviously I would only jump at a much smaller distance; 200 feet was a little bit too much for anyone, let alone for me!

So the next day, Maddo, Gav, and Jack, coached me on how to do a jump. Even though I was riding again, I hadn't jumped a ramp yet, especially one that was so big. That day, Maddo was jumping 200 feet, so he drew quite the crowd from the traffic going by. When he was finished, the boys dragged the ramp right in to a gap of about 25 feet from the up ramp to the down ramp. This wasn't a huge gap for the professionals, but it was big enough for the average rider.

As a crowd gathered, I became very nervous. The last time I was in this position was when I had my accident, so a lot of old emotions and dark memories started to get in the way of my judgment and focus. I did a few test runs, but the more I tried talking myself into doing it, the more I got nervous, and the boys could tell.

Maddo rode over to me and asked what was up. I told him what I felt and what was going through my mind, so he shut the jump down straight away. He said that maybe it was too soon, so we rode back to the truck and got changed. I felt like I really let the boys down as well as let myself down, even though they were the ones who told me to pack up.

I said to them as we were getting changed, "I think if the crowd wasn't here, I would have been fine."

Gav said, "Well Wood boy, there's always tomorrow. The ramp won't get pulled down until late morning, so if you're up for it, go for it tomorrow."

I was happy with that. That night, we went out for a few quiet beers and had an early night.

The next morning, Maddo and Gav kicked open my door around 6:30 a.m. and said, "Righto boy, you gonna do this or what?"

I laughed and said, "Clearly boys, I've been waiting for you to wake up!"

We had a feast of a breakfast cooked by Kazza, and then we went down to the jump. The boys talked me through it. Maddo showed me on his bike what speed to do, so after my first speed test run, I decided I to commit to the next speed run. Maddo, Gav, and Jack stood at the bottom of the ramp watching me from the tray of Gav's F250. I went to the start of the run-in and imagined the jump. This was my moment of truth! I didn't spend time thinking too much about it, because if I did that, then all of my fears and doubts would rise up and I would probably pull the plug on doing it again. Without hesitation, I went off! Soon after I clicked into second gear, I aimed straight for the ramp and pushed past the point of no return. I focused on getting over to the other side, and committed in full trust into not just myself, but also into what Maddo had just taught me.

As I went up the ramp, I kept my mind focused and did not fall into the second-guessing mindset. I thought about the moment that I left the ramp on my snowboard, which contributed to the accident that nearly took my life, but it was only for a split second in the back of mind, and then it was gone! *Whooosh!* I was quickly in the air and no sooner I landed on the other side. I made it! I landed it perfectly! As soon as I landed, Maddo let off some fireworks he had, and the boys ran to me to congratulate me, but I didn't stop. I let out a huge scream of joy, a few other choice words, and I went straight past them. I didn't want to stop then!

I jumped about 12 more times, and then finally I had to stop. They needed to pull the ramp down to transport it back to Melbourne the next day. The boys were so excited for me; they had just witnessed me overcome a huge fear and hurdle a milestone in not just my journey of recovery, but in my entire life. I put every bit of self-doubt and doubt from everyone who said I couldn't do this to the side, and I overcame it all.

That night we went out for dinner to celebrate. Maddo had to fly to Melbourne the next morning and I was going to go in one of the convoy cars for the five- or six-hour journey back to Melbourne too.

I jokingly said to Gav and Jack, "We should ride the Harleys to Melbourne."

Gav just said, "Alright boy, you can."

And Jack said, "Well, I'm up for a ride so let's do it."

That was it then—it was settled! At 4:30 a.m. the next morning, the convoy of trucks and cars left, and Jack and I were on the Harleys. This truly was going to be a weekend that I would not forget.

Around dawn, just after 5 a.m. we jumped on the Harleys and took off to Melbourne. It was summer, but the air was still pretty fresh at that early time of the morning. There were no excuses—I committed to this ride, so I had to follow through. An hour into the ride, Jack pulled into the petrol station to fill up his Harley, so I followed him in.

Just as I went to stop, something was going on with my right leg and I couldn't feel it properly. It felt like it went to sleep, and I didn't realize just how much it had until I tried to move it and I couldn't. I yelled out to Jack to tell him what was happening, and he braced himself. I did a lap of the petrol station and came back in with Jack ready. Somehow, he caught me just in time and helped me get off.

Right then and there, I thought, *Fuck! I've got five more hours of road ahead of me. Have I bitten off more than I can chew?*

But I had no choice. The rest of the convoy was way ahead since we left and hour after them. So I walked around, warmed up my leg, and Jack waited by my side until I was able to continue riding he then jumped on his bike and caught up to me.

After that little scare, I made sure to move my legs around to keep them from falling asleep. It was such an amazing ride through the Australian outback, and we watched the sunrise over our beautiful land! We took our time until we were about an hour out of Melbourne. Then once we got on the freeway we tried to catch up with the boys. We got to the outskirts of the city to a main fuel stop at Calder Park, and the boys had just arrived there.

Gav was so pumped for me.

He said once again, "Geez wood boy, I could see your grin a mile away! Well done, mate. You've defiantly ticked off a few boxes this weekend!"

I still fondly think back to that weekend and recollect what those boys did for me. They helped me not only do new things in my life, but they also helped me to overcome huge fears.

I can't describe the feeling of riding side by side with a mate in the Aussie outback and riding through our amazing countryside. We watched the sun come over the hills and it was the most awesome feeling of total freedom I have ever experienced.

That weekend gave me back a huge part of my life, and I continued to get back more and more of my life as the days, months, and years went by.

## Maddo Josh and Jack at Quick Fix

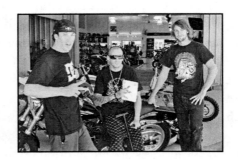

# Chapter 9

# Spreading the Word

## Impossible really means, "I'm possible."

I have been fortunate enough to get into Motivational Speaking, or Inspirational Speaking. I didn't think I would be very good at speaking in front of crowds, but mum had a lot of faith in me that I could do it and do it well.

I enrolled in a media course that offered classes in motivational speaking. They taught me all the techniques that are associated with speaking in front of groups of people. The classes ran for one two-hour evening once each week. I didn't enjoy being there at all, because I didn't think I was going to be any good. The funny thing was that I received really positive feedback from my tutor and others in the class.

I obviously picked up a thing or two from the course, because not long after I finished I found work to speak to different groups. The audiences varied from schools, corporate, small businesses, and insurance and risk workshops.

With so many twists and turns throughout my story, I had a lot of wide-ranging experiences that I could speak about, so each presentation was different. Many people seemed to connect with my message on many levels. I got fantastic feedback, on many occasions I noticed people in the audience crying, I always knew I had touched them when I experienced this. My talks were really just about life: goal setting, prioritizing what is important, using visualization techniques to create a positive future, believing that anything is possible, and of course, the motto I live by: Never Give Up!

Securing continual speaking engagements in Australia was tough,

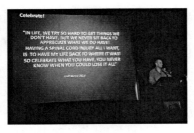

especially since I didn't have promotional material, like a book, DVDs, or consistently facilitated workshop seminar courses, which would have given me more credibility. It was so frustrating because there were many people who were excited about my story. Some were extremely supportive and I received fantastic feedback and most times standing ovations after many of my talks, but the speaking circuit prospects for me dried up and I decided to drop it for a while.

Then, Amelia came into my life and she encouraged me to get back on the speaking circuit and start mentoring people, so I rethought the whole motivational arena and the opportunities I would have if I was involved at that level. With help from Amelia and mum, I reworked my presentation and made my stories a little more edgy and raw, which took them to a whole new level.

I felt much more confident in getting back into the speaking circuit.

I liked the thought of getting back into speaking to large audiences again. I worked with someone who helped me with publicity, and between us all, we sourced out people and groups that I could mentor and motivate.

## From Amelia's Journal

### It's talk time!

Josh regained his confidence and decided to do more talks. Throughout June and July Josh spoke around Australia. They were mostly day trips but when they required an overnight stay I would travel with him and I loved travelling with him. It was like having lots of 'mini honeymoons!'

Basically, I took my speaking format right back to the beginning and kept it true to me. It was just me telling my story: about my accident, what inspires me, and what keeps my focused on moving forward. I think that's what makes my talks so powerful. It's not just about a message, but it's a story—my story, my life. It's about where I was in my life—a regular healthy 18-year-old guy living my passion, which was snowboarding and a bit of motor cross, and then having that life taken away in a split second to be replaced with a much different life—one that was filled with injury, many restrictions, adversities, limitations, and constant pain.

It was informational and educational, and it included the following:
- How I got movement back.
- How I walked again.
- The "mind tools" that I used to keep myself focused and positive.

And I especially stated how I kept refusing to give in and accept that this was all I had! I always emphasized the importance of celebrating any achieved goals. I also pushed the message of keeping things simple.

I presented that strong message along with the visual aspect of the groups seeing me in person. This was the basis of what I used when I spoke to audiences, and especially when I mentored someone.

Since I live and breathe my own story, it's a much more powerful statement than it would be if I just ran off a bunch of statistics and a series of diagrams about what happens when people get a spinal cord injury. I am my message! People relate with it and they connect to it in a different way than they would if I was just presenting them with a bunch of medical reports and pictures.

## From Amelia's Journal

### Right on purpose!

It was important for Josh to get back into his public and motivational speaking because it gave him purpose. It reassured him that what he has done is amazing and inspiring.

I have seen just how Josh connects to everybody when he speaks, even people without a Spinal Cord Injury benefit from what Josh has to say. They are able to connect it to some part of their own life story so he has a much broader demographic of people that he appeals to and that's because his message is not just about how he physically rewired his body but about the power of the brain and will power, reinforcing to people that they can do whatever they put their mind to and that the impossible is in fact possible with the right balance.

*Actually I like that! 'The impossible is in fact possible!' Great title for a motivational talk!*

My talks run between 45 minutes to just over an hour, depending on which group I am presenting to. The content is pretty full-on most of the time but that's just me. I tend to not edit and censor myself. My story isn't pretty. It's grueling at times and full of emotion, which is why I tell people who have a spinal cord injury and their family, or whoever wants me to come and speak to the person with the injury, that my message isn't supposed to be taken lightly.

Sure, it's an inspiring and hopeful message, but it's designed to push boundaries and limits, to get the audience to think outside of the box, and to push the message of the power of the human mind to overcome almost anything.

My mentoring is on a whole different level.

I don't rush in and see people as soon as they are injured. They need to be in an open mindset and not be closed down with fear and uncertainty.

What people don't understand about me is that I'm blatantly honest, raw, and to the point. I tell it like it is. I don't make fancy promises or give people false hope, but I have certainly been accused of that from the medical professionals on numerous occasions. But that accusation is just bullshit because that's not who I am.

People don't always like what I have to say and sometimes they can be afraid of the truth. I'm not afraid of the truth—in fact, I'm the kind of person that I'd rather be told the truth, even if it feels rotten hearing it. I'd rather deal with that than have anyone tell me "fairy floss" facts just to make me feel good. That's how I survived when I was in hospital. I didn't want to be told half-truths or be misled. I would rather be told what people think of me, or tell me what I've done wrong, because then I know what to fix, and I'm a big believer in telling people what they need to fix.

My injury and my recovery generated a lot of interest, especially through the exposure I received after I was interviewed on a primetime Australian Current Affairs television show. I backed that up with commercial radio interviews and then approached organizations that I thought would be interested in my story and would like to have me come out and do a talk.

Slowly I began to build up a presence and people started to hear about me.

People wrote to me and contacted me because they heard my story and they saw that anything is possible when they have absolute determination and will power combined with the correct mindset to change their situation. They relate it to their own lives in some way and that's fine because I'm happy for people to approach me or make contact with me, and I try and help them in any way that I can.

What I don't do is individually target someone or source anyone out.

I would never say, "Oh a new spinal cord injury. I'm going to write to them and fish them out!"

That just won't happen! I always make sure the contact comes from them first. If it's an injury, then the desire to change it or fix it has to come from that person, and they also have to want to do the work and put the effort in themselves, because no one wants to really fix anything if it's just handed to them. If they think it's easy and people want it like that, then when they see me and hear what I have to say, they realize it's not so easy.

## One of my biggest inspirations

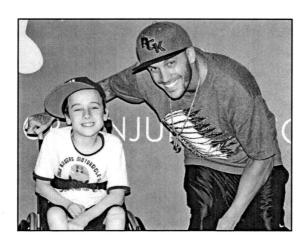

## From Amelia's Journal

### Twice Born is born!

People mould the "Twice Born" Josh Wood theory to all different aspects of their life, from weight loss to relationship problems, school bullying and even a child dealing with the fact that both of his parents have cancer. I have seen how welcoming people are to Josh's message, it makes sense to them and I think the fact that Josh breaks it all down and encourages people to keep it simple and not complicate it has a greater appeal.

They see it in Josh; he is very much an example of what he speaks about how little by little the greater goal is achieved. I've said this before—it's about making sure people don't set unrealistic goals and the importance to celebrate each time they conquer a goal, and that in itself will motivate the individual.

I've had people say to me countless times, "Oh, you're so lucky with what you've done."

I don't think I am lucky. I only think I'm lucky in the sense that I have the most amazing and incredibly supportive close network of family and friends around me.

My mum never gave up on me and she made sure I didn't give up either. When I hit that low point right at the very beginning—when I was so brutally told that I was a complete quadriplegic and would never walk again—I wanted to die. Mum wasn't having it and she got the fighting spirit in me going and there was no going back after that. Mum was certainly the catalyst in flicking the switch on in my head and I never thought of giving up like that again.

My wife Amelia has been a tower of love, strength, and support to me. She goes through it with me everyday, and that's why we don't spend more than day apart from each other. She sees everything I have to go through just to get me up in the morning and on with my day.

Even with all the constant support around me from Amelia, mum, and her two sisters, the decision to do all the hard work had to come from me. The only person that was going to do the work and get me walking again was myself.

# Kay

As I have mentioned many times, it has taken a global village to get Josh to where he is today. The village has consisted of his wife Amelia; my sisters, my late mother Dottie, and other family members; and friends, not just from all over Australia but also throughout America, Bali, and Ireland. There have been all sorts of medical and alternative practitioners and healers along our journey as well: our amazing, dedicated, and committed A-team.

Then there was me there supporting him all the way through his recovery. I knew my son and I knew what he was capable of; in my wildest dreams after all these years, I didn't realize that my son had such a relentless will to recover. No matter what happened, he always got back on the road to recovery. I look back now and realize how naïve we were that we never researched the injury until these last few years.

As for me, there's that saying: If you're no good to yourself, you're no good to anyone else. It took me a long time in this journey to realize that I needed to heal too.

There are many things that I learned from the experience of Josh's injury. I learned that I had to keep myself well, positive, strong, and in good shape mentally, emotionally, and physically to be able to keep helping Josh.

Two of the most important lessons that I learned were to be positively selfish, to take me-time, and the power of detachment.

At first I really struggled with doing anything for myself because Josh had my whole undivided attention 24/7. In those early days, I wondered how we were going to manage financially, so I arranged to sell everything we had, and I went without sleep, I didn't eat properly, and my work and business suffered. Josh's accident happened during my busiest week of the year. It was the only week of the past 11 1/2 months of work that would bring me my most valuable payday: the bringing in of the deals, the final negotiating sales and finance contracts—yet all that was forgotten!

I still had to make calls to my clients, but I just couldn't leave the hospital, so I relied on friends and family to help me when they just turned up. Our friend Jenny contacted my clients, spent hours in my office making calls, sending emails, and sending faxes.

Life around Josh still had to go on. I wanted to be there for Josh

100 percent, but I also needed to do everything else. In those first few weeks, I absorbed so much information that my brain ached and my heart ached. My heart really did break the moment we were told the news of Josh's accident. That pain caused me to have enormous pressure in my chest for months.

I couldn't eat, I couldn't sleep, I couldn't stop, and I was on the go around the clock. The one emotion that I can say ruled my world was fear—total fear. Well, it doesn't take a scientist to work it out that this wasn't going to be sustainable for me, and if anything happened to me, what would happen to Josh? I had to balance it out and I had to take care of myself along the way.

I had to make time for a haircut, sauna, spa, and I had to just spend some time pampering myself. It was amazing how rejuvenated I felt afterwards—don't underestimate the power of what a one- or two-hour time out does. Over the years, I mentored many families and especially the mums. I always emphasize the importance of taking me-time to them.

About year three post-accident, I spent 18 months taking therapy sessions. I learned to mourn Josh's change of destiny, the loss of his life as it was planned, and mourn the complete change in my life plan. Going to therapy was cleansing, enlightening, and empowering. I paid someone a lot of money to listen to my ramblings, but it was well worth every dollar spent!

I was an avid reader but I felt too stressed to read, so activities that mentally challenged me really helped me through those dark early days and weeks.

The second lesson I learned was about detachment. I learned how to let things go and to not dwell on what can't be controlled. I detached from people and things that hurt or stressed me. I personally believe that the skill of detachment was the most valuable thing that I learned from this devastating period of our lives, especially in those early days.

I still practice both of these skills: me-time and detachment. They get easier with time.

What our support village did to help Josh get his life back was a combined effort of all our experience. What Josh did to get his life back was never give up and he believed his body would heal and he would walk. I now feel we can comment on it and say what worked for us since it is no longer guess work. We worked it out ourselves with the help of some amazing people. The one thing that still causes me great frustration is the attitude of his doctors. They didn't get Josh's prognosis wrong; they know where he has come from. Many years ago one of his doctors stated in a forum of peers that Josh has achieved something that in all his years he had never experienced anyone in Australia achieving—the fact that he walked after such a devastating injury.

His words were, "we need to learn from this young man."

That was in the first 12 months after Josh's accident. After 13 years we are still waiting for the western medical profession, especially the doctors in that hospital, to take the time to learn from Josh. That would make such a difference to all those newly injured.

Even if I had all the help and assistance from the best therapists, practitioners, and chiropractors, I still absolutely needed more than anything and anyone else to believe it in myself. I say "in" myself because there is a big difference between just believing something and then taking that belief internally.

When I send people to see therapists and chiropractors and such, I say to them that it's good to see these people, but they shouldn't think for a minute that they are going to just lie there and get all the work done for them, and then just get up and walk out. It just doesn't happen that way. People with injuries like mine have to believe that the therapy is working on them as well as inside them. They have to believe that their body can heal, because if they don't believe it, then it won't work. They have to physically believe that they can feel their body healing. It is difficult and most people don't like difficult—they won't do difficult.

People write to me and say, "Oh, I've heard about your story and what you've done. It's amazing that you walked in five months. Tell me what your secrets are."

And I think, well, *There are no secrets. I just wasn't a victim. I never entered that victim mentality; my accident was my own fault so there wasn't anyone else or anything else that could take the blame.*

It was all me, but I was not going to play the role of victim. I don't believe I have the right to complain about my injury when there are people worse off than me but they are happy and living their lives.

My mate Bronte was a perfect example of someone with a spinal cord injury who didn't let it stop him living his life, and he didn't play the victim role either. During the times when Bronte was in a wheelchair, I didn't see the chair because he wasn't any different character-wise than he was before his accident. He was just this amazing person and he was amazing to be around. That was inspiring to me.

So after the first week of my accident, I decided, *Fuck it. I've got to do something about this. I can't just lay here dwelling on what could have or should have been.*

In those early frightening days, yes I missed snowboarding, yes I missed motor cross, yes I missed being able to walk, and yes I missed my freedom more than anyone, but I knew that if I thought about that all the time, then nothing would get better.

I thought, *Okay I have to live now. I need to live and move forward from here, so what the hell do I have to do to do that? I have to keep it simple. I have to get my toes moving, so we'll start with that.*

I started to do all the visualization. Straight after my accident, Paula the psychic taught me meditation, visualization, and how to go deep into it and I practiced it all over and over again. Eventually, I became quite good at it and I had very good results with those techniques. Sometimes it was extremely hard, and at times I had to visualize something for six months before it worked. My attitude and my belief was that I couldn't move on until I achieved the result, so I could never skip a goal. If I did, I wouldn't proceed to the next level.

When people come to me for mentoring, I tell them that it's not going to happen overnight. It may not even happen for them for two years. I am convinced that the ones who walk again or gain improvement over the original diagnosis are the ones that never give up! They are prepared to do the hard work to chip away at it every day.

It's not just about walking; it's about getting a piece of your life back one way or another. It could simply mean gaining some independence to do things for yourself and not need assistance, or it could be as little as getting movement back in a finger, or being able to scratch your own nose. That's the one thing I missed doing the most—scratching my own nose. When I got that nagging itch in my nose or anywhere else on my body, no one can scratch it the same way I could. These are all the things we took for granted before this injury and now they meant so much more. The freedom to scratch my own nose! Who would of thought it would mean so much?

The ones who are committed to getting in deep with their visualization and get results from it never sit there and think, *I've done it five times over and nothing has happened.*

It could take a million times. I was the kind of person who would rather try a million times than try just once and then give up.

## From Amelia's Journal

### Completing the impossible!

Josh 'died' on so many levels when he hit the road at the ski resort on June 25th 2000 just 18 years old!
- Physically, everything he had died!
- Emotionally he died!
- Psychologically he died!
- Socially he died!
- And for a brief minute—his body died!

That's when he had his rebirth—his second opportunity at life—hence, his 'Twice Born' experience into the physical shell of an 18 year old but he had to equal that in ability and in some cases, Josh had less than a new born baby has ability to do things.
- He couldn't even cough because his diaphragm was paralyzed!
- Breathing was no longer an automatic response.
- He had no use of his bladder or bowel.
- The use of his limbs was gone!

Emotionally, he gained power to put all the sadness aside and overcome the want to commit suicide and using all he could psychologically and spiritually so he was 'Twice Born' in every sense on every level.

He found the power to take on the impossible! (Here's another motivational talk!!!) Even when he was constantly told "best case scenario, you will be in an electric wheelchair with little movement in your right arm," he wouldn't settle for that, he found the power to never give up and the power to never give in. He never gave in to the demons in his head when he lay motionless, just a head in a hospital bed, alone with his thoughts, 18 years old and unable to protect himself.

I once saw this cartoon strip where these two guys digging horizontally through a tunnel underground. The digger on the top tunnel is digging away with his pick and he's going hell for leather pacing along. He has this manic expression on his face and he has cleared just over half way. The digger in the tunnel below him is digging at a steadier pace but has dug further along his tunnel, about three quarters of the way along. The next frame of the cartoon has the top digger still digging along at his crazy pace but he's still got miles to go. The bottom digger has stopped digging, turned around, and is walking back to the beginning of the tunnel looking very defeated.

The irony is that the top digger, who has the crazy face and is digging frantically with his pick, thinks he is just about to break through and claim his reward. The bottom digger who has given up and decided to walk back to the beginning of the tunnel only had one miniscule area of rock to dig through to a treasure trove of jewels and riches. He never knew how close he was to breaking through and getting the rewards because he gave up.

I think that cartoon perfectly describes this injury. If spinal cord injured people stop "digging," then they don't know how close they are to getting that next bit back. That's how I look at it, and that's as simple as it has to be.

The doctors will only fix their patients to a certain point. Mum always said that the doctors would fix me but they wouldn't heal me, and she was absolutely right. The only person that could heal me was me.

It probably would have been easier if I said, "Well, I've been dealt this card, so I'm just going to learn how to do my sports and live my life in a wheelchair."

That way, I would have known in my life that this is what it is and where it's going—that I would just do everything from the chair, and that's okay for those that do! But I couldn't do that; even though I didn't know what I was going to get back or even if I was ever going to get anything back at all, I still fought every day to learn how to walk and find out if there could be something more for me than spending my life in a wheelchair.

I still only have 5 percent cord function at C6 and C7, so as far as spinal cord injury goes, 95 percent is a very high percentage of non- functioning cord. If the cord were severed, that would be entirely a different story.

Since I still had some strand of cord still intact, my theory was, *Why can't I get movement back?*

In my case, there was still some cord connection, so I believed there was something to work with.

## From Amelia's journal

### Odds? What odds?

He has overcome such defining odds! He was given only a 3% chance of any sort of recovery! He was left with only 5% use of his spinal cord. Given those sorts of odds, it would be perfectly understandable if Josh made no progression with his recovery!

But Josh is gutsy! And combined with the power of his determination, motivation, mind, spirit and belief, Josh brought all that and worked it into his treatment and recovery and that was the power that got him to complete the impossible! (There's the talking circuit title again!)

What Josh has achieved is remarkable! It definitely became the catalyst of his post injury journey and everything combined has accumulated into the 'Twice Born' experience. It is such a powerful message and his message just has to be heard.

So if people in wheelchairs saw me and heard my story, would they want to know more? If so, then I am a good example of what is possible because I did it. I was able to go from a wheelchair, to standing, to walking with a stick, to walking un-aided. This isn't anything against people in wheelchairs; unfortunately, in a lot of cases, most cord injury people don't get the option to get recovery and movement back because their cord has been so badly damaged. I'm referring to myself and to the people who have a better chance of getting something back.

I have seen with my own eyes the people who have had major cord damage, classed as "complete" and still get some new function back. My friend Barney Miller, who is a higher-level injury than mine, barely did a thing in the first few years of his injury. Then, a spark ignited in him and now Barney can stand, and he's also able to surf and travel everywhere. I was lucky enough to also be there the night he got down on one knee (with the help of two Project Walk trainers) and asked his soul mate Kate to marry him. It was definitely one of the most moving nights I have witnessed. I look up to Barney and his attitude to life and how he takes it on. I don't think I have ever seen his face without a smile, unless he has his "concentration face" on at Project Walk.

There are so many others who inspire me with their own personal recovery. They are all examples of patients who have also been told by the medical professionals that it was impossible for them to walk and they would be wheelchair bound. Barney, Bronte, and I are all examples of proving these medical professionals wrong. We all learned to stand, walk, and even get on with our lives.

The human body and mind is capable of doing miraculous things. There have been countless documented incidents of the human body achieving something that has been said was not medically or physically possible.

A classic example of this is the first person to break the four-minute mile. The two athletes that did it first, Roger Bannister the English athlete and then Australian athlete John Landy, said it best:

> *"Breaking the four-minute mile barrier was first achieved on May 6, 1954, by Roger Bannister.*
>
> *"It was a sense of relief," says Bannister, recalling the momentous event more than 50 years later. "There was a mystique, a belief that it couldn't be done, but I think it was more of a psychological barrier than a physical barrier." John Landy, who broke Bannister's record with a 3 minute 58 second finish only six weeks later, argues otherwise. "It has nothing to do with psychology," he says. "It was just a matter of having the right runners at the right level of training and the right set of circumstances."*

I agree with both statements.

I believe that recovery from a spinal cord injury is a combination and application of all these things—overcoming the psychological barrier, the physical barrier (if there is any functioning cord), and having the right person with the right level of training and circumstance. As I've stated before, it is not about walking; it is about never giving up on some sort of recovery and believing that it is possible. Anything is possible with belief, determination, and never giving up, and that's up to each individual spinal cord injured person to come to their own conclusions in regards to their injury, what they accept, and what they believe they will and won't get back.

When I mentor people, they often don't see the progress they make, so I always encourage them to film everything. I sometimes regret that

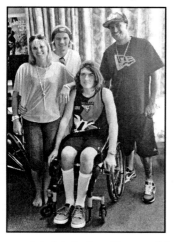

I didn't film myself in the first nine years of my injury. I didn't see myself walk until two years ago; I never let a camera near me. My biggest regret is that I never got to do that. I never got to see my own progress and how far I've come and people look at me now and they say, "You're fine," but medically speaking, After all these years, I still present as a complete quadriplegic. I walk and I'm grateful for that, and I don't let that gratitude go easy, but if I sent my MRIs to any surgeon in the world, they will think I'm in an electric wheelchair. No way would they would think that I'm walking.

I knew that if I saw myself unable to walk, then that visual image would stay in my head, and that would be the picture my mind would hold onto. But I was still Josh. I was just broken, so I didn't want any photos taken of me that would show me how bad I walked or how disabled I looked, because I knew if I looked disabled, that would stay in my head. In my eyes, I just thought that I was injured. That's how I looked at it; I kept it simple.

I didn't want to see any film that showed me struggling because I didn't want to see my arms not working or my legs wobbling.

I remember the first time I saw myself on film and I thought, *This guy should be in a wheelchair.*

That was three or four years ago, so if I thought that back then, I might not have regained the movement and mobility I did because I was too vulnerable back then. It's a different story these days; now I watch it and say that I'll fix it because I'm stronger now. I look at my videos now in the same way that I used to when I watched footage of myself snowboarding or riding motorbikes. I would film myself in action so that I could watch it later and see what I was doing wrong, and I would know where to change it.

It works the same way in reverse: if I was in a photo with the wheelchair, then I made sure I couldn't see the wheelchair in the photo because I didn't want my brain to have a relationship with the chair.

When I started working with Bronte, I asked him, "When you go to bed and you wake up in the morning, what's the first thing you do? What's the first thing you see?"

And he said, "My wheelchair."

And I said, "Well, piss it off, get rid of it, push it down the other end of the bed so you can't see it."

The more the brain sees the wheelchair, the more it's going to think it needs it. My brain is so used to me walking like this, that it's more of a mental thing now. I know my legs can do a hell of a lot more stuff. I've snowboarded since my accident, I can ride a dirt bike, I've run a couple of times, and I've walked at Project Walk.

During one of my training sessions at Project Walk, I looked at Amelia and she was crying, and I said to her, "Why are you crying?"

And she said, "Because you are walking normal."

For that moment, my brain forgot how my body had grown used to walking. It relaxed and I was fine, but then it went, "no, this is wrong," and I reverted back to my own walking style.

I understand why it happens and I recognize that it's more of a mental aspect with me. That's why I am working more on a mental level now.

With the mentoring I try not to bog people down too much; I say things like, "Keep it simple, don't let it all get on top of you, don't miss the things that you miss."

They usually say, "That's easy for you to say."

And I tell them it's not, because I loved snowboarding; that was my life—I loved motor cross and BMX, I loved being outside, being able to run, jump fences, and climb trees. I was an active kid, but I knew the reality was that I couldn't keep doing all that.

So I started an internal question and answer dialogue with myself; I would ask, *How am I going to get back to that? Well, I'm not going to dwell on that. I'm going to move forward.'*

This is something I tell everyone, whether it is in my talks or my mentoring. It is vitally important to get the self-talk right as much as it is to get the self-visual right. You can't afford to sabotage yourself with negative self-talk and feel sorry for yourself. It's easy to be a victim. I'm not being harsh; I've got mates who are in wheelchairs and they have a life as good as what they had before whatever it was that put them in the chair.

People say to me, "How do you stay so positive?"

Well, I see people who are much worse off than me and they are happy every day, so I don't have the right to be anything else.

In those early days when I was in the hospital, it was about mentally keeping strong. If my mates were coming to see me and they were going to cry or be upset in front of me, then I didn't want them there. Mum warned everyone that if they cried in front of me, then she would throw them out of the hospital. You have to move on. You have to acknowledge that whatever happened has happened, and just get on with it.

My mum says, "Okay it's done, over, delete, move on."

And that's how I've always been. That's my coping mechanism; that's exactly what I needed.

Don't get me wrong, I have some terrible days when I feel like throwing it all in and giving up. There are times when I feel completely done in, but never long enough to get stuck. I'm definitely not perfect; I'm only human, and for some reason, I just never give up. There is something embedded in me that snaps me out of it—whether it takes me minutes, hours, or even a day.

At the start I didn't know what techniques or treatments would work or what wouldn't work so I just kept trying different things. Over the years, I have found out so much about me, and what does and doesn't work. Now I might try something different and I know that if I think it's not going to work, then I'll just move on and try something else. I might come back to it a year later and try it then, and if I get the same result, then it's "over-delete-move on!"

Initially, in those early days, I did so much visualization that I slept for four or five hours after I did it. That was doing half an hour of concentrated visualization. My body was already fatigued from the injury and it was early days. To the people I mentor, I explain two visualizations I did that worked well for me in the beginning. I have already discussed these techniques earlier in the book, but I feel that they are so important for recovery and getting movement back, so I'll briefly restate the technique for both:

With puppeteer visualization, I closed my eyes and imagined a video camera going through my body, starting from my brain, and then going down to my legs. Once I had the visual of my feet (from the inside, looking at the ligaments, tendons, and muscles), I then imagined pulling on the ligaments, just like a puppeteer pulls the strings that are attached to the puppet to make it move. Remember that I chose to work on my big toe on my left foot, because I'm a lefty. I also started with my toes because they were the weakest part since they were so far away from the initial point of my injury.

With the charts visualization, I kept my eyes open. I looked at the male body anatomy chart in front of me and I studied the formation of the muscles: what they looked like, the length of them, where they began and ended in the body structure. Then, when I had the visual of a specific muscle, I knew where to squeeze to get movement.

To summarize it perfectly, Amelia said, "You can't connect internally anymore. You have to connect externally."

I had an AFL (Australian Football League) player contact me once. He had problems with his bones. He wasn't meant to play in the AFL again, but one of his team's coaches heard about me and brought me in to see him. I spent two hours with him and all I did was tell him my story; where I started from, what I did, and the results I achieved. I reminded him that he still had his team, family, and friends who believed in him, so he had to believe it himself. Most importantly, he had to have self-belief that he could heal himself and he needed to know that no one else was going to do that for him.

He went and played his comeback AFL game a year later after he was told he'd never play again. That's why I look at every individual and their situation as unique to them and I choose very carefully what I say. I find that I can't go wrong if I just tell them my story.

I still go through pain and I still have bladder and bowel problems. My bladder function came back for about six months, but because my urethra got so used to using a catheter, it collapsed. I still live through the sensory pains and the phantom pains. I'm never comfortable, and I've never been comfortable in my life since my accident. I tell my listeners about this in my mentoring sessions. Some people see me standing and looking okay, so they hear what they want to hear.

Others listen and say, "That's awesome."

When I do my talks, people see me stand in front of them. In their eyes, I look healed. I make sure that I remind them that I still have all those phantom pains and neurogenic pains. I still feel like my whole body is on fire 24/7 and a lot of other things I go through but can't be seen from the outside. People only see what's presented on the outside, but there's a hell of a lot more going on inside.

I really enjoy all the talks I do, especially my one-on-one mentoring. I get to show others who are having a tough life that they can overcome any obstacles that life throws at them. They can get breakthroughs and improve the quality of their life. When the body is injured, it can heal itself. Sometimes I talk to two or three hundred people at one time. If I can get through to only one person in that audience and it makes a difference in their life, then it's worth it.

My story is simple. I'm all about I *can!* I'm not interested *I can't!*

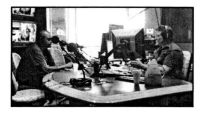

# Chapter 10

# No Labels!

## In my mindset, I never allowed myself to be labeled.

Total recovery was my number one priority. I refused to believe anything less was possible.

When my medical team labeled me, it was the one thing that I battled with the most, especially in those early scary days. Obviously I had an injury that they had seen countless times before—they were the experts are after all—they classed me as being a C5, C6, C7, T1 complete quadriplegic at that time I was admitted—that's what they told my mum and dad.

Even though I was 18-years-old, I was still a kid in many aspects. So as a kid, I had no clue what that realistically meant. What was a "complete quadriplegic?" There was a label straight away of who I was! I wasn't Josh Wood anymore. I was a quadriplegic!

In my mind—whether it was denial, or whether it was just me being my strong-headed self—I just kept on telling myself, "No, no I'm not a complete quadriplegic. I'm Josh Wood and I'm broken, but I will put myself back together. I'm broken but I will walk again."

I kept this mindset; I never called myself a quadriplegic. I have never let myself fall in that trap of being labeled. I knew that as soon as I labeled myself as a quadriplegic or gave myself any other label that made a similar statement like, "This is it, this is what I am now," or "This is what my life is going to be," then in my mind that would feel like I was giving up.

I have nothing against people who do call themselves quadriplegics or paraplegics, or who are confined to a wheelchair; it was just my personal self and my choice that I never wanted to label myself something that I believed I wasn't. I already placed in my mindset that I was only broken and my way of thinking was that if something is broken, then it can be fixed. I made myself think that I had just broken every single bone in my body, and I had to repair them.

## Kay

Our words were always carefully chosen. Josh wasn't disabled; he was injured. He wasn't having therapy; he was having recovery. We treated his injury as an injury, so the words were always couched around this activity!

In my opinion, a huge part of the recovery process for someone suffering a spinal cord injury is focusing their minds on treating the injury as an injury and not as a disability, and working through a process of injury recovery.

I am becoming more and more certain that the stronger the will is to recover, the more chance you have at experiencing recovery, but nothing is easy, and sometimes the recovery is so subtle it is easily missed.

I believe that bringing in the alternative practitioners and therapies right from the start of my accident made all the difference in my recovery. It wasn't only the healing work they did on me that helped in my recovery, but it was also the techniques they taught me so that I could work towards fixing myself. After the "attitude" the medical team gave me, there was going to be nothing conventional at how I was going to fix my broken body and walk again. It was all going to be alternative modalities, because I felt that all the alternative therapists had my back. They were always encouraging and supportive.

The most important point was that I trusted them. This was the biggest difference for me between the two types of practitioners; I trusted my alternative healers a lot more than I trusted my medical team. I felt that the medical team wasn't in my corner. They never gave me hope; they were determined to make me accept their label for me . It frustrated them that I was so defiant that I didn't accept their label. I questioned their attitude and behaviour towards me. They gave me no confidence, no benefit of the doubt, and they would dismiss every movement as nothing more than an involuntary spasm. They had a negative justification for every small piece of progress I made.

What they didn't count on or understand was I had a greater positive justification that at 18 years of age. I was going to walk and live my life just the same as I would if I didn't have this accident. I set my mind on fixing myself and I was going to walk. Nothing and no one was going to have me believe or accept anything less.

One positive aspect from my medical team was the work my surgeons did to repair my neck. The repair was textbook accurate with minimal scaring and they properly rebuilt my vertebrae and removed the floating splinters and chunks of bone. They were great at mending me, but not great at healing me with recovery after the surgery.

I understand that they have to cover themselves as far as telling their patients the worst-case scenarios, but when that is the only scenario they offer, then I think that's pretty poor. It's not about telling someone the probabilities of whether they will or won't walk again. It's more to the point that no one has a right to play God and determine someone else's future, especially when they don't really know what that future really is.

Their views and opinions were all speculative as far as I was concerned, because in theory, with the extent of my injury, I should have not been able to walk, whereas in practicality, I did walk.

## Kay

Keeping Josh positive was crucial, yet so often the hospital system worked against him! We learned to not trust anyone in the medical team, even though in the beginning we had no idea what to do.

We just trusted our gut instincts, and if we weren't happy with something that the medical staff were doing to Josh or if they were being unduly rough, then we would speak up and we challenge the nurses or doctors. We did have excellent nurses and doctors; they just didn't have the same care that we wanted for Josh. In their eyes he was a C5, C6, C7, T1 complete; in our eyes he was our loved one.

We soon became very good at assessing what was good, what was bad, what was working, and what wasn't working.

One day when we were standing beside Josh's bed, one of the nurses came in and she threw Josh's medical charts on his legs. I was in total shock of her action and I asked her why she just threw the charts on his legs.

She answered, "Well it doesn't matter, he can't feel his legs anyway."

Well, I can assure you she will never do that again.

My injury was just as hard on my family and friends as it was on me. It was probably even harder on them because they saw me in pain a lot of the time. They saw my frustration at constantly being told by my medical team that I wouldn't walk again, and they saw me struggle to get movement back.

As much as they wanted to help me any way they could, I knew it was all up to me and that I had to take control of my recovery. I had to just keep looking forward and never look back. That's probably why I am the way I am now—determined and to the point. If something or someone happens to pull me back into being a victim or into doubting myself, then I will cut what or whoever that is out of my life and move forward.

I had to take that hard line because I was in survival mode. From that point, that's where I worked hard, and I did a lot of visualization and goal setting and never labeled myself.

## Kay

One thing I was determined to do for Josh, whether he was in a chair, in bed, or on crutches, was to keep up his appearance. Josh was always particular about his hair—how it was cut and styled.

The hospital and rehab had a barber, but the styling was pretty basic, so I arranged for my hairdresser to come in to the hospital to cut Josh's hair. He came in two or three times during the time Josh was there, and he travelled about an hour each way. He never accepted any money from me. It never ceased to amaze me how caring so many people were.

Another thing that Josh was always fussy about was his clothes. He always wanted to look good, and he did always look smart. I remember a few days after Josh was admitted to the acute spinal unit, the nurses told me they were getting him up the next day so they asked me if I could get some cheap Target brand tracksuit pants and some moccasins or slippers.

I asked, "Why do we needed moccasins?"

They answered, "Well, he won't need shoes anymore!"

"So why moccasins though?" I questioned because I was still a bit confused at that request.

"Well, they are comfortable and his feet will swell."

I left the hospital with Josh's mate Dutchy and we went to the outlets nearby and I bought Josh some designer brand tracksuit pants and a pair of skate shoes that were two sizes too big. I wasn't about to show up at the hospital with cheap trackies and moccasins. I'm sure that if I did, then Josh would have believed I had given up on him.

Once I left rehab and hospital, I tried to get back into as normal of a life as possible. I went back to the same gym that I used to train at with Dutchy. I still had to go to an out-patients' rehab centre nearby, but I only went to four or five sessions and quickly got over it. The rehab centre was such a depressing place and now that I was out of all that, I never wanted to go back.

So I started to train back in the gym. The more I did normal gym work, the quicker my mind and body developed. My personal trainer helped me transfer onto the machines so I could do the exercise as normal as possible. I could have done them all from the chair and it would have been much easier, but that would have meant my butt would clock up more hours in the chair, so I did it the hard way. I trained nearly every day and at least two times a week I was with my PT (personal trainer). On the days that I wasn't training with my PT, I devoted my time to healing sessions from my alternative healers.

One of the reasons I went to alternative healers is because they made me think. They got my brain thinking of ways to improve and heal. That's where I got my strength from because I was proactive in my recovery, not passive.

My alternative health team was the ones who encouraged me and believed 100 percent in my recovery. I gathered such a diverse cross-section of alternative health practitioners, but combined they each addressed the different areas of my healing and recovery. As I have always said, this might not work for everyone, but it certainly worked for me.

## This was my team

### The 'A' Recovery team:
- Simon: Chiropractor, my mentor, my friend (ongoing team member)
- Paula: Spiritual Healer, Crystals, Meditation, Visualization
- Isabel: Massage Therapist— Chakra alignment, Chi energy
- Uschi: Cranial Sacral therapist (USA 2011-2012; she will be an ongoing team member when I return to the USA)

### And the rest of the team:
- Jackie: Reflexologist
- Bing: Acupuncturist
- Ben: Personal Trainer (2001-2005)
- Dr Graeme B: my personal Medical General Practitioner (ongoing team member)
- Micco: Hypnotherapist (USA 2012; I will continue to work with him in the USA)

There were several other great alternative healers that came into my life all throughout my recovery journey. They continued to show up just at the right time to offer the right kind of technique that I needed at that particular stage of my recovery.

My weeks were also filled with two sessions a week with Simon, one or two sessions with Isabel, and one session a week with Bing. Communicating with Bing wasn't an issue. Even though she couldn't speak much English, we managed to connect and we understood each other. Up until then, I hated needles, but this was part of my recovery journey and I had to do a lot of things that I hated and would never have tried before. Bing was so good at what she did and she gave me such amazing results that I got past my hatred of needles. I didn't mind being a human pincushion for those couple of hours each week.

She came over to the house once a week to work on me there for up to two hours. The regular acupuncture sessions helped so much with my circulation, sensation, and they also helped to reduce the spasms in my legs. I actually really enjoyed the sessions with her. It matched up well with the work that Paula, Isabel, and Simon did with me. They all knew each other and they all worked together on me and each used their specialty technique. Every now and then, Bing massaged me. I felt so relaxed when she worked on me, and with all the consistent and frequent sessions I had, my body started to wake up bit-by-bit.

# Kay

We were fortunate to have such a great group of dedicated alternative professionals involved in Josh's recovery process. Through our chiropractor Simon Floreani, we were introduced to Jackie who practiced reflexology. Jackie worked for Simon in his practice. Once Josh was admitted to the acute spinal unit, Jackie came in on Saturday nights and worked her magic on Josh's feet. She worked with Josh for about two hours always behind closed curtains. We brought in local take-away food; Chinese, Thai, or whatever we felt like, and we (except for Josh) enjoyed a glass of wine from cardboard cups and had great chats while she worked away. It was such a pleasure to be with positive people who genuinely cared about Josh and were always positive about his recovery.

Jackie came in several times while Josh was in hospital. She never expected to be paid for her time, and the hospital was a long drive from where she lived. We were extremely grateful for her care and enthusiasm. Reflexology is an ancient Eastern healing process, which is primarily practiced on the feet and soles of the feet, but it is a concentrated healing process that deals with nearly every bodily function and organ depending on the area of the foot being worked on. It is fascinating how the soles of our feet control so much of our bodily functions and organs.

Whilst we are advocates of this healing technique, as it surely assisted Josh's well-being, we are only are here to say what worked for him. Any other spinal cord injured individuals should always do their own research before using anyone to work with.

We had one doctor who was totally on our side and a huge help to me, especially during those scary early days—Dr. Graeme B. Graeme had been Josh's doctor for several years before his accident. Graeme was more than our doctor— he was our friend. When

Josh had the accident, Graeme wasn't involved due to the specialist nature of the injury. He gave me his mobile phone number, so when I was concerned or confused, I would call him at anytime and just ask him what he thought. Graeme totally supported our alternative approach; he knew Josh and he knew Josh was smart enough to integrate what he needed. Graeme is still our doctor today and we are both very grateful for his love and support.

We were fortunate that we had these people in our network, in our lives, or someone who knew us that referred them to see Josh. Of course, it was always Josh's decision whether he wanted to have them involved in his recovery or not; he always had the decision control.

In those early recovery days, my schedule was pretty full and getting my life back was now my full-time job. I still socialized with my mates, but there was no chance of partying excessively or hard drinking—I didn't have time for that. I didn't drink any alcohol for about 18 months. I was too focused on keeping my body as clean as possible, giving my body love, and giving my body a chance to heal.

## Kay

Just before Josh had his accident, he used to work at Crown Casino (Melbourne) in the Sports Bar—he was a barman. He loved his job there. One Saturday he decided he wanted to go to see his old work mates. Josh dressed as he normally would; the only thing different was he was in the chair. He usually crossed one leg over the other and he really just looked like he was sitting in a lounge chair.

As we came up from the car park into the casino, Josh became really frustrated because people were staring at him. I just kept trying to calm him down. It was so hard; he looked terrific, although he had lost a lot of weight.

Getting through the Saturday night crowds inside the Casino was a nightmare, but we finally arrived at the Sports Bar and he enjoyed a short break as he spent some time with his old friends there.

In a small way, this was him beginning the journey of regaining his old life.

Another thing I did, which always got a reaction out of people, was when I sat in a wheelchair with one of my legs crossed over the other. I did that everywhere I went in the chair. I always shifted my body about and crossed one of my legs over the top of the other so I looked the same as everybody else. I did that because I wanted to show that I could sit just like able-bodied people sit—that I wasn't any different when I was seated, yet people always stared at me and tried to figure out how could I be in a wheelchair but still be sitting like an able-bodied person with my legs crossed.

I think that out of all the places I socialized at, the venues I felt I had the most reactions and stares from people were the at regular nightclubs and at the Casino.

## Kay

Josh didn't want his life defined by his chair. As he became more confident, he started to go out to nightclubs, always surrounded by his mates who respected his independence but looked out for him. His friends were so protective and caring that it made my heart swell with happiness.

There were many stories of strangers who made snide remarks to Josh in the chair. On several occasions, the boys used the chair as a weapon. One night, it was actually thrown down a set a stairs directed at someone who had made a disparaging remark about Josh. I was always relieved when he arrived home after one of the nights out. Even though these outings didn't always run smoothly, they were very important to attend with his friends because it meant that Josh was getting his independence and life back.

The most challenging and confrontational venues for me to socialize in were nightclubs. Young drunken idiots gave me bad looks.

Some would say, "What the hell are you doing in a nightclub? Shouldn't you be at home? What's wrong with you?"

Or they defiantly stood in front of my path and stopped me from being able to get past them. More than a few surprised drunks learned their lesson in how to treat people a little better, to not be judgmental, and to keep their lame comments to themselves. Their first fundamental mistake was to assume that I was a weak pushover who would take shit from anyone just because I was in a wheelchair.

After everything I had been through, I wasn't going to put up with individuals with a "hero" mentality or take any type of bullshit from them, nor were my mates. I never went out looking for trouble because I had been through enough hell already. So others started it, but I always finished it, whether I shut them down verbally or physically. Most times my mates reacted quicker than I would, because they were always very protective of me and always kept an eye on me.

One Sunday night, a few of the boys and I went to a local bar. It was a pretty big place. At this time, I had just started to walk a lot more and use my chair less. As I sat down, a security guard came over to me and said, "Mate, I'm going to have to confiscate those elbow crutches from you."

I didn't know if he serious or not, so I said, "Is this a joke?"

And he said, "They could be used as a weapon if a fight breaks out so I'm going to have to keep them with me."

I began to see that he was serious so I asked, "What if a fight breaks out and I need to get out of the way? What if there's a fire? How am I supposed to get out?"

He leaned over to me and said in a sarcastic voice, "Well, I'll make sure I get them to you."

I just said "Yeah, I'm sure I will be your first priority when something goes down. So I guess every time I need to go to the bathroom, the bar or go outside, I'll have to call out to you so you can bring my crutches over?"

He said, "Guess so, mate."

He lifted up my crutches and walked off with them. I waited until he got back to his post and as soon as he put my crutches down next to him, I started another full round of back-and-forth questions and answers.

I yelled out, "Oi mate, I need my crutches."

"Why?"

"I need to go to the bar."

He made a big huff sound and then brought them back to me. I went to the bar and my friend carried my drink back to the table because I couldn't since my hands where full holding onto both crutches. As soon as I sat down, the security guard came across, grabbed the crutches, and off he went.

Once he got back to his post, I called out again, "Oi mate, need my crutches."

"Why?"

"Need to use the bathroom."

He rolled his eyes, picked up my crutches and brought them back over to me and said, "Mate, you doing this to piss me off?"

And I said, "Pretty much! You've taken away my ability to walk and have independence. Clearly you didn't take my feelings or situation into consideration, so I'm going to take away your ability to do the job you were hired to do—so yes!"

After a few more choice words, he gave up and let me keep my crutches next to me. The fact that I had to go through all that still makes me angry, but that's a small drop in the stupidity pond I went through.

One of the other frustrations for mum and I was the way some people reacted to me in the chair. They talked to mum instead of to me and have a whole conversation with mum right in front of me. It was like I was invisible.

Mum would just say to them, "Talk to Josh, there is nothing wrong with his mind."

Or, if people weren't ignoring me, then they would either talk loudly or slowly at me. It was like they thought that because I was in a wheelchair, I might have some kind of mental disability.

Then there were the people who just stared at me as if there was something weird about me. I hated it when they stared. Mum used to say they were not used to people in wheelchairs being dressed normally. It was important to me to look and dress as I did before my accident. I was still Josh and just because I was in a chair, it didn't change how I wanted to dress and show who I was. I guess people always saw the chair first and then me. That's why every time the minute I arrived at the place we had gone to, whether it was a restaurant, club, or somebody's home, and I got settled, I transferred to a normal chair and moved the wheelchair out of site.

## Kay

One thing that Josh always insisted on and did every time was transfer to a normal chair and discretely move the wheelchair out of sight. This occurred whether we were at home, in a restaurant or out visiting. We always made sure that the chair was put away. When he went to bed at night, he pushed the chair away down to the end of the bed. He didn't want to wake up in the morning and have the chair be the first thing he saw.

In the beginning, this was difficult because he had to move down his bed to get in it in the morning. He also hated having the chair in the car. He always put it in the trunk because he just didn't want to see it.

Most of the time when I went out, 90 percent of the people were always nice to me and helpful. If it was a tight place for me to wheel or walk through, people shifted across or moved out of the way, but every so often there were always a few people in the crowd who gave me a hard time.

Parking my car has been the single most annoying situation I have had to contend with. I sometimes got sniggering looks from people if I pulled up in my car and parked in a disabled car park. People stopped and watch me. They saw me get out, stand, walk around my car holding onto it, and get my wheelchair out of the back. They didn't have to say anything because the looks on their faces said it all. I knew what they were thinking because I had it said to me many times before.

"Is he putting on an act? Why is he like that? Does he really need a wheelchair if he is walking?"

If they only knew what I had been through and gained, what I had lost and may never get back, would they really still be so opinionated? That saying, "Never judge a book by its cover" is very relatable for me because I'm that book!

# Kay

One of the more positive labels that Josh was given was "Rudder Boy." by John G.

John and Dana, who joined our family for Christmas celebrations in 2000, gave Josh this crown. Just after our Melbourne Christmas celebrations, Josh, his then girlfriend, John, Dana and I went to Noosa Heads on the Sunshine Coast in Queensland for 10 days.

It was Josh's first flight since his accident and the doctors were worried about clots forming, so Josh had to have injections in his stomach before flying.

It was also our first flight using a wheelchair. Josh had just got his new chair; it was electric blue with carbon fibre mag wheels. Even his wheelchair had to look cool. We had just received it after waiting for several months for it to come over from America.

Noosa was beautiful as always, and although it was the rainy season, the weather was quite good. Josh was keen to get back in the water again and feel the freedom that being in the water gave him. There is a lagoon on the north side of Noosa at the end of the village. We went down there and John just kept on encouraging him to get in the water. There was a boat moored out a short distance from the shore and John challenged Josh to swim to the boat and touch the rudder. Always up for a challenge, Josh swam out to it and back to the shore, and then out to the boat again.

John started calling Josh "Rudder Boy" after this—it was such a fun time in a year that had been so challenging. We enjoyed lots of laughs and fun times on that trip; it was what we all needed.

The Christmas after my accident, mum's good friends Dana and her husband John flew over to Australia from America to share the holiday with us and help me with my recovery. They had been a huge help and support, not just for me, but also for mum. John came to the gym with me and swam in the pool. He encouraged me to try something new every day, to set goals, and keep a journal. This was something I was not good at, but John always reminded me to keep at it, so that I could see the progress I made.

We also went up to Noosa for a holiday with them, which we all enjoyed. There is no holiday from this injury even on a holiday, so we always did things that kept me moving and active, whether it was John and Dana meeting me at the hotel pool in the mornings and doing some morning walking and training in the pool, or hitting the hotel gym and doing a workout.

John and Dana told me that they had a plan for me to head over to America about six months after our Noosa holiday for more recovery treatment in order to help me retain my Chi energy. They generously offered to financially fund the time I was over there. All mum had to fund me for was my airfares. At that time, she had nearly a million frequent flyer points, so we set the dates and mum booked me into first class on United Airlines. The only condition was that I had to stick to my training program and diary entries. This offer from Dana and John was a huge motivational goal for me, so I did exactly what they asked.

Once they went home to America, I got right into my program. I stuck to my training; I ate right, and I kept my mind and body focused. I was so absorbed in my daily trainings and routine that I didn't notice the days and months flying by.

John and Dana stayed true to their word, and six months later I was in California. No sooner had I landed in America, that they had me in their car and we travelled to Southern California to introduce me to another alternative healer, Mark, to further help with my recovery. He was a Chi Master who had done a lot of healing work on them.

I liked Mark as soon as I met him. I felt really comfortable for him to work on me. I didn't know what to expect, but if Dana and John knew him well, and they had him do healing work on them, and recommended him to me, then that was good enough for me. He worked on me for two long and intense hours and he focused on and in restoring my Chi energy. At the time, I walked using two elbow crutches, but only around our home—rarely outside unless it was a close walk. Within two sessions of working with this Chi Master, he had me walking down his hall, down his stairs, and then out his front door and down his drive way! It wasn't a fast or graceful walk by any stretch of the imagination, but I was vertical and moving forward and that was better than anyone could have imagined.

This blew my mind! All the pain and hard work was truly paying off in such a short amount of time. In only a year, I had come so far and gained so much back. There weren't any miracles; it was just sheer determination and hard work. It was the best gift that Dana and John could have given me. I stayed with them for about 6 weeks in LA and Colorado. It was a time of great learning and healing for me. Mum and I were very grateful for their help.

I came home and continued with all the training and programs I had been doing with John in the States. I was still learning to understand my body and the many changes that occurred after the accident, and what it could and couldn't do. One thing I couldn't do after my accident was sweat, so I decided to start using the sauna. In my mind, that was the quickest way to regenerate sweating, because it was a struggle for me, especially in summer. The first time I tried the sauna, I spent 20 minutes in it and came out bone dry, but I persisted. After a few weeks, my body started sweating from below my injury. Within a month, even my legs started to sweat. What I found interesting was that if I had researched sweating, I would have read that most people with a cord injury never regain the ability to sweat. Luckily I never researched it!

## Kay

In those early days, going out in the wheelchair was really a challenge. Josh suffered with leg spasms, so when he was agitated, they got worse. Josh described his legs as "crazy legs," but over time he learned to control the spasms and used them to aid his recovery.

One night I was enjoying a concert at a club. I was having a great time, listing to the bands, relaxing, and enjoying myself. I was sitting down on a bar stool and after a while my left leg was jumping, which was a sign that either my leg had fallen asleep or that something else was happening to my legs.

Just as I looked down, my mate said, "Woody, your jeans are on fire!"

They quickly threw water over my legs and put out the flames. Someone must have flicked their lit cigarette and it landed in the crease of my jeans. We all had a laugh and didn't really think that much of it until the next morning, when I was about to transfer into the shower. I looked down and I noticed my left ankle was really swollen; as I looked closer,

I realized that the cigarette had burnt two deep holes in my leg, one the size of someone's small finger nail and the other the size of a bottle lid. I couldn't believe it! I couldn't feel it at all. It made me realize that I had to be so much more careful about my legs and to make sure that I always checked them if I was near smokers or anything hot. It was something I never even really thought about before, especially being burnt like that, but I never forgot that lesson. Because of my poor circulation, the burns took several weeks to heal. I refused to go to the doctors and chose to heal it myself.

Having a Spinal Cord Injury creates a whole different meaning to planning a day out. Being away from the safety of home was and still can be a challenge. For some reason, that's when things go wrong and they go wrong in the worst possible way. I always have to plan everything to the last detail and make sure I have everything I need. Whether it's me being on the boat all day and making sure I have my things I need so I can go to the toilet, or making sure I'm hydrated if I'm in the sun or if I am staying overnight at someone's house. I wasn't concerned about my legs or ability to get around unless it had to do with parking in the city, distance, hills, or weather. All of these were things I never had to stress about before, but with SCI, I had to take all those factors into consideration.

Above all the things I contend with on a daily basis, what always plagued me the most were my bladder and bowl problems. It has taken years of practice, failures, and success to feel confident about leaving the safety of home. I'm still tested with this daily function from time to time.

A few years ago, I had three or four accidents that really destroyed my confidence. When I say accident, I mean the worst possible and demeaning kind of accident.

Once while I was at a night club, I knew I had to use my bowels, but the first bathroom was filthy and had no toilet paper so I had to go down stairs and across a dance floor through the crowd and to the back of the club where the other toilet was. I held on the whole time, knowing I had a very small window of time before I was going to be in trouble. As soon as I got to the toilet door, it was too late! It literally happened. One of my ultimate fears, aside from it happening on a plane; this was number two in more ways than one. I just shit my pants in a nightclub, and what was worse was that the bathroom was at the back of the club and it was closing time. I was horrified, so I cleaned up as much as I could but it was still quite bad.

I managed to wait until most people were out of the club and then I made my escape. The problem was that I had a few drinks so I couldn't drive home. Originally I was going to stay at my mate's house and leave my car in the car park but after what had just happened, I definitely didn't want to sleep at anyone else's house, so I went to my car. Luckily I had some wipes that were from a fast food shop, so I cleaned myself up as good as I could and I had to sleep in my car the way I was. This broke me down in so many ways—the fact it happened at a club, the fact I had to sleep in my car and still not feel clean—it broke my confidence in so many ways and it was so demeaning.

A week or two passed since then, and I visited a mate who lived about and hour from my home. We had a great dinner and we spent some time just hanging about. Time was getting on and I had an hour's drive home ahead of me so I said goodnight and headed off.

During the drive home, I started feeling unwell in my stomach. I was too far from his house to turn back and I knew there was a petrol station not far down the road, so I did all I could do to hold on until I got there. The petrol station was in sight but it was too late—the unthinkable happened again. I was gutted.

I just thought, *Why me? Why now? What the hell have I done to deserve this? I'm so over this fucking injury and not being able to control anything! This hasn't happened to me since I was in hospital and now it has happened twice in a matter of weeks! Is my body shutting down?*

Those two accidents really destroyed my confidence. I was too scared to go anywhere or do anything after these accidents but I knew I had to snap out of it. There was no way I was going to become a hermit and shelter myself; I had to get my confidence back. I had to change my mindset and think about what was going on inside and why.

So I changed my diet and I made sure that if I was going out anywhere, then I would go to the toilet first and just try to make sure I have no chance of this happening again. I had to learn from this; something good had to come out of it. I always made sure that I would try my hardest to learn from every experience or accident. It was tough, and it still gets me down, but I learned from it. I can see the funny side in the situation now and I joke about it.

I often talk about my issues and turn them into humour. I always thought that people around me judged my situation or thoughtless of me until recently, when I realized that those were my own thoughts and issues. I realized that when I spoke about these issues, people actually thought better of me, because I could still hold my head up high and not let it dampen my spirit.

Back in 2011, we went out to celebrate Amelia's birthday with friends. Laslo and his girlfriend Sharah, Amelia, and I had arrived at a club. We walked through the crowd to get to the bar and order some drinks. As we made our way through the club, Laslo heard a group of guys make a derogatory comment about me. Laslo let it go; he didn't want our night to be ruined and he didn't want me to hear what the guys said, so he left it alone. As we got to the bar, the girls ordered the drinks. My back was against the bar as I talked to Laslo and I could see he was upset about something.

I asked him, "What's up?"

He said it was nothing to worry about. There were about four or five guys right near him that where staring at us, so I asked Laslo again what was going on.

He replied, "They were talking shit about you and bagging the way you walk."

I laughed and said, "Ha ha, they must be jealous that I have my own original style and they are all the same."

Laslo laughed. It was obvious that these guys were acting like big heroes as they carried on laughing and pointing at us.

Las then said to me, "Josh, one of them said to his mate, 'what's a hot chick like that doing with a cripple?'"

Before I could come back with a response to Laslo, the group of guys walked over to us at the bar. They obviously thought that we wouldn't stand up for ourselves since they outnumbered us.

One of them said to us, "You guys got a problem?"

And Laslo replied, "No but you guys will if you keep talking shit about my mate and getting in my face."

They exchanged a few words with Laslo, and I thought, Ahh damn, here we go.

The next minute, the loud mouth bloke lined me up, took a cheap shot, hit me, and split my lip. Before he got a chance to know what happened after hitting me, Laslo knocked him out cold. Another idiot came out of nowhere and bottled Las across the top of his head, but that didn't faze him. Laslo then knocked out two others, one after another. I somehow managed to push Amelia out of the way and also retaliate back to land one hit, which broke one idiot's nose.

Before we knew it, security was on top of us and the drunken idiots were getting dragged out of the club. It wasn't until they were gone and we were still standing at the bar that we realized how bad Laslo's head was. It was cut open from being bottled. We also realized then how split my lip was, but it wasn't too much to worry about. After a drink, we decided to head off and get Laslo's split head sorted out and my split lip looked at.

I do not condone fighting. I never ever look for fights because I don't know who is out there and what they are capable of, so I don't know what's going to happen. This is the frustrating part of my recovery. Here we were just minding our own business while celebrating my wife's birthday with friends, and it took one idiot group of heroes to change our night dramatically. Thankfully, none of us were hurt too badly. I can't say the same for the troublemakers. It was unfortunate for Laslo that he got hurt, but he wasn't fazed because all he cared about was that I was fine and he hoped Amelia's birthday wasn't ruined.

I try not to go out to clubs much these days; it's too hard for me to get around, especially with no cane to keep my balance. Although walking without my cane was my goal, I am still getting used to it after all these years so it's not as easy for me anymore. Walking unaided takes so much concentration to keep myself balanced while making sure I land each step. Sometimes, my right foot decides to drop to early, which causes me to trip and fall. Throw a fast moving crowd and loud thumping noises into the mix and it just throws me off. That is my reality; until someone lives in my shoes, they won't understand.

I chose to walk and never rely on a chair, so I can't complain, but it still gets frustrating.

I wish I could carry all the heavy shopping bags up our steep driveway. Or, when the dogs get sick, such as Montana hurting her leg recently, Amelia had to carry her, but I should be able to. But wishing and getting upset doesn't make things happen, so I use it as motivation. I turn it into a goal and add it into my training régime.

Don't get me wrong—it does get me down, sometimes to breaking point, but after feeling sorry for myself for an hour or so, I realize the problem hasn't been fixed, so I find a way to manage, change my situations, or motivate myself to make it possible in the future.

Recently, Amelia and I had a little getaway weekend at a spot we both love and we spent as much time chilling out as possible. We were at the caravan park at the river and I needed to go up to the store, which was a short walk, but it's difficult because the road has a loose rock surface. It was a really hot day and I usually don't stay out in the sun for too long in case my body warms up too much and gets dehydrated. So I went to jump into my car and drive up. Amelia asked me where I was going.

When I told her I was just going to the shop in the caravan park, she said, "Are you serious? Why don't you walk?"

I was about to reply, "I can't be bothered."

But before I said that, I thought about my situation. I realized after all I had been through the challenges of wanting to walk again, getting so far in my recovery, and the many people with similar injuries that would love to do what I can do, that even if it's a struggle, I had no justifiable answer, so I said, "Okay, let's go."

Before I knew it, we were off and walking to the store. It was a lot harder walking on my own. I had some sketchy moments along the way, but I did it! It was such a small thing, but the power and confidence it gave me was awesome. From then on, I always challenged myself and at least tried. What's the worst that can happen? I get tired? Sore? Trip over?

## Kay

The journey I had with Josh, from the moment of his accident to his hospitalization and rehabilitation, to his road to recovery and beyond that, to his progress, triumphs, tribulations, marriage to his soul mate, to his further recovery, setbacks, and now success, he has given me the greatest sorrow mixed with the greatest joy of my life. If someone told me 13 years ago how dramatically my life and Josh's life were about to change, I would have said they were crazy. Life throws curve balls—there's no doubt about that. As one of the chapter headings in this book, "When Life Gives You Lemons, Squeeze With All You've Got!" Well, we have both squeezed with every ounce of fibre in us. I have seen first-hand the strength of the human spirit, but I have also seen the worst of it.

While many people have been amazingly supportive, encouraging, and helpful, some people have been extremely detrimental and insensitive towards Josh. As his mother, it has both infuriated me and broken my heart to see the negative and sometimes hostile treatment that Josh has encountered because of his injury. People fear what they do not understand, and I certainly had my share of fear along the way.

The first time we heard the term "SCI" (spinal cord injury) was 16 March 2011. We had to ask what it meant! Josh and I walked away from the SCI community on the 11 November 2000, the day he left the rehab facility. We were both sick and tired of the negativity and the "You can't do this" attitude. So, although mentoring many SCI people over the years, back in the beginning we operated so far out of traditional recovery techniques and we just did our own thing until we heard about Project Walk.

That state of the art facility, the trainers, the programs; all of it made such a difference in Josh's recovery. We already laid down the foundation for Josh's recovery with the amazing Recovery Team we had built around Josh. Every healer and practitioner who worked with Josh knew him or knew of him. They were either friends of ours, friends of friends, associates of our small Recovery A-team of three, or recommended by them. Josh was completely trusting and open to what each and every one of them did for him.

I wish to emphasize this is what worked for us, everyone we had work with Josh, we trusted and they were extremely gifted. This is not an endorsement for psychics, healers, masseurs, hypnotherapists, personal trainers, chiropractors, reflexologists, acupuncturists, sacral cranial therapists, or any other alternative modality we sought help from.

We never worked with anyone we didn't feel confident in. In all cases, with the exception of our chiropractor, not one of our healers knew about spinal cord injury or its implications. Our journey with Josh's spinal cord injury was in 2000, not 2013.

Those with SCI should do their own research and build their own team, whether it's from conventional or unconventional methods.

Josh was prepared to do whatever it took to heal, recover, and walk again. He was also prepared to have no labels placed on him.

This is the first time that our story has ever been written, but it is a story that always needed to be told!

# Chapter 11

# No Excuses!

## Even the best excuse is still an excuse.

"No Excuses" started after Amelia and I got back from America. We spent the last four months in California attending Project Walk, catching up with some of my Aussie mates who lived in California at that time, and we were introduced to some amazing alternative healers. These last four months had changed my life on so many levels. A lot of good things happened while Amelia, mum, and I were there, and some amazing people came into my life and took my recovery journey to a whole new level of intensity and breakthroughs. I couldn't wait to get back home and see my dogs, family, and mates, and show everyone the progress I had made.

Four months was the longest amount of time that I had been away from my dogs Montana and Thor. To say we missed them is a huge understatement. When Amelia and I arrived home and they saw us, they were so excited and we were just as excited to see them. We didn't let them go, nor have we since we have been home. Montana and Thor are pretty much with us 24/7. They are as much a part of our life as they can be. The only time they are not with us is when we are out socializing at night, but even then we have been known to sneak them into hotels!

We came back at the perfect time of year. It was the start of summer, so Christmas was coming up and we were ready to have some fun, go up to the river, and relax. It was the time of year for us to do our summer activities, like catch up with friends, have our BBQs, go out in the boats on the river, go down to the local tavern, have a feast of great food, and drink my favourite beer.

After being home for two weeks, I already started to slip again. When I was in America, I had structure and a training routine that I followed every day and now that I was home, I slipped back into having no drive to maintain my health and fitness routine, and I developed bad habits of not doing my training. I had no gym to train in, so that only added to my lack of motivation to train. I was not eating healthily and I ate too much BBQ food. I was also spending too much time just hanging about catching up with friends. The only good thing was that my appetite for partying was far from my thoughts. I knew I would quickly undo all the great progress I made in America, so I had to put some structure and routine back into my life straight away.

One of Amelia's friends found out about a Personal Trainer who lived just around the corner from where we lived. Amelia asked her friend if he would be available to do some training with me and look after my health and fitness needs. He said that I should come to the gym where he trained so that we could have a chat and see if we could work out something to help me.

So I met with the Personal Trainer, who was named Jason. We had a great chat and hit it off really well, really quickly. He came up with the idea of helping me with training. I could then see what he could do for me with his off-the-wall training programs, using boxing, pushing and pulling heavy weights, and getting my leg strength back, along with my core body strength, which is what I still needed.

About a week later, we started training together. I told Jason at our first meeting that my finances were at an all-time low due to huge costs of attending Project Walk for four months and having to organize everything towards my upcoming wedding with Amelia.

I didn't like to do things and get it all one way. I try to give back and have it all equal and balanced, so I presented Jason with the idea of doing the "No Excuses Project." Basically, what it involved was not making any excuses. Most people have their goals, but they also place all these excuses and conditions on starting their fitness and health programs such as, "We're going to wait until after New Years Eve," or, "We'll have some fun over Christmas, eat lots of food and drink a bit of alcohol, and then we'll fix it next year."

I wanted to show Jason my commitment to him and the "No Excuses

Project," so I started the program, which was a basic, straight to the point outlook on looking after myself and remaining focused on what's truly important. I designed it to be an example of everything I said and did throughout my own training and recovery programs. This new project, or chapter, meant eating totally healthy food and definitely no booze.

Amelia filmed all our training sessions to hopefully inspire anyone to achieve or set new goals for themselves. She collected the diet tips that Jason provided for me each week, and then she edited the information of all the things we did together to create a motivational video from it.

I started training with Jason about three weeks before Christmas and we trained three or four times a week. It was really intensive training—just the type I absolutely love and have no trouble committing to. I also committed to a healthy eating regime. I didn't drink any alcohol and I only ate clean healthy food. Even Christmas day and New Year's Eve didn't escape the new health kick! We didn't have anything that was detrimental. We only drank soda waters and plain water. I wanted to prove to people that it's not living in the future, but it's living in the now and being committed to the process, and to not make up any excuses to get out of doing the hard work.

This new way of well-being was a really easy thing for me to do and to sustain. I really loved it and I got so much out of it—a fitter, healthier, and stronger body, better sleep, longer sustained energy levels, and I was a lot happier mentally and emotionally. I was in a really good place.

The wedding was only twelve weeks away and Amelia did her own fitness and health program. She is such a fitness fanatic that her enthusiasm and commitment motivates me. Her motivation was one of biggest reasons I decided that I wanted to fix the health and fitness aspects of my life. I didn't want to come to the realization that I had enough time to change things but didn't fix anything, or that I tried to turn things around when it was only three weeks away, and I had wasted the nine weeks prior.

In the lead up couple of weeks to our wedding, I still consistently trained three or four times a week with Jason. I also trained by myself, even if I was just at the gym stretching out. It felt good just to get down there into that fitness environment. I used the rowing machine a lot in my routine, rowing a kilometre a day and swimming a kilometre a day as well. On the alternate days when I didn't use the rowing machine, I mixed it up with other exercises and fitness training machines so that I didn't get bored and my body became used to working out in the same way. If I mixed it up, then my body stayed stimulated and I stayed focused.

We filmed everything I did in training and posted it once a week on various social network sites. We did this to motivate other people and to prove that there is no time like the present to fix things in life.

I had absolutely no money in the bank at that time and I could have used every excuse possible—I didn't have any money, I couldn't see my friends as much, I just wanted to cut loose for a little bit—but I decided that I wasn't going to use any of those excuses. I was going to stick to my guns and fix my health as priority number one!

One thing I do lack is core strength, and because of that, I was never able to get rid of the excess body fat on my stomach. It wasn't a lot but it was enough to bother me. It's really hard for me to burn it off with swimming and cycling because I can't put in the distance, time, and intensity needed to shift it.

Jason helped me address it by changing my diet. He devised some diet plans for me to follow. The first thing he helped me with was structuring my food. Simple things, like no concentrated carbs after 3 p.m. was a huge thing for me. I struggle with knowing which foods I should be eating as well as with cooking the healthy food, so it was good having Jason and Amelia there to help guide me. They both made it a lot easier. Other people don't always have those benefits, but luckily for me I did and I shared it with others who may not have the knowledge around them.

It is tough to stick to those types of foods and eating routines. I love meat, I love eating charcoal chicken and lots of other foods like pizza, but with the new eating plan, I was taught to eat in moderation and I had your one "cheat" meal once a week. If I had it after 7 p.m. then I tried to have it with water to break it down in my system—no soft drinks or carbonated drinks. It really helped a lot with my food intake. I don't always eat as clean as I should, but I have my food structured, so I am much better now.

I have even managed to drop off about three or four kilograms of weight off my stomach and I gained it in other ways like in muscle mass. Losing that weight in six weeks helped me and benefitted me enormously.

Even though I didn't get to my exact body weight that I wanted, the changes that I made on a physical and health level made a huge difference. More importantly, I was able to spread the message to people that it's all about being committed to now and not later on.

Another thing we did with "No Excuses" was we made sure that it was adaptable for a lot of other people. It wasn't just concentrated on putting me in the spotlight. We tried to incorporate structure, other training programs, and healthy eating regimes for people that were injured or in wheelchairs so that we could help them in the recovery journey.

Many of us don't have that cardio time, or energy capacity, or fitness levels where we can go for runs, or go for long walks and other cardio options, so that's where food becomes really important. People tend to think that it's all about the training, but the diet is the biggest capital that helps you with losing your weight and losing it in the right spots. It is not just about losing weight—if someone is injured and in hospital, diet is such a huge factor for wellness, especially for recovery. Injured people shouldn't eat junk food, fizzy drinks, energy drinks, or anything that makes their system sluggish, or anything that is hard for the body to process.

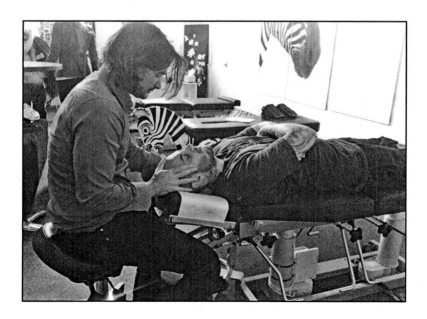

The correct diet helped with my core strength, especially because there is so much lack of movement in my body. It was amazing what eating the right food, getting the right balance and portions did. All that made a huge difference in what we did. The right training routines and healthy foods definitely helped gain more strength in my body.

Everything I experienced, learned, and incorporated into my life over the past months have changed my life in the most dramatic and beneficial ways. This is the new improved way of life for me. Everything in and around my life now follows one rule and has one message: "To keep things simple."

I think the problem I had was when I got myself into a tailspin, because I got really stressed about not having any money, not feeling fit and healthy, and also just from thinking about things I didn't have.

One thing that I talk about every time in my talks is that I tell people, "Stop thinking about things you don't have and start thinking about things you do have."

Once I started actually listening to myself, I realized there were a lot of things I needed to fix. I needed to do this without trying extremely hard to fix them, or trying to push them along a bit too much too quickly. Once I sat back, enjoyed life a little, and did simple things that made me happy, then everything started to come to me a bit quicker and a bit easier. My fitness was coming along a bit better, and so was my overall health. I put the word out without trying to push it too much. I motivated people and myself at the same time.

I was motivated and encouraged by people who would write into me and say, "Oh wow, I didn't know you could do that, that's amazing."

They came back to me and told me about the sort of things they were doing and that motivated me as well. It made me want to rise to the next level and move forward. I wanted to show my family, friends, and the people who were becoming aware of who I am, that I'm still not giving up and I never will give up no matter what. There have been plenty of times where I could have had the excuse of why I gave up, but I never did.

I look back at the last 13 years of my life and what I have achieved. I just think that it was my nature to get things done and go beyond what even I think I am capable of. It's just who I am, and I have always had that stubborn determination to never to give up and never give in. I always thought that if I went that little bit extra, then I never knew what I might get back. In a way I'm forced to never give up. If I give up or get too lazy, I fall apart, and it's much harder to bounce back these days. I've been dealt these cards and I can either get lazy and complacent about it or I can kick my own arse and keep moving and achieving so that I can have a better future.

After having the freedom of a fully functioning healthy body for 18 years and losing it all and going back to being like a baby and not being able to do a single thing for myself, then to fight every hurdle and wall, break through them and to continue fighting after 13 years—I feel like I can use my story as an example for people to base their own goals and motivation from.

For the first 10 years after my accident, I never put my story out there on any social media site. I never ever posted videos or photos, and when people asked me, "What have you done to your leg?" I always brushed off what I had been through and just say, "Agh, I've got a screwed ankle from an old injury."

I didn't like to talk about my accident or recovery because I didn't want people to feel sorry for me or think that I was trying to get sympathy. It's not just about spinal cord injury; I use my injury and recovery as an example, but it's really just about everyone's journey through life. It's about how people can pick themselves up when they get knocked down and how they keep moving forward.

My message is about realizing the gift we have and to not abuse it, whether it's the gift and freedom of a fully functioning body, the gift of being in a solid loving relationship, or the gift to having the courage to take on life head first and never look back. It's to know that even if there seems to be an impossible obstacle that you can't see around, with determination and the sheer will to better the self, anyone can indeed make it possible to get around it and live strong.

It comes down to how hard we are willing to push our comfort zone, our mind, our body, our beliefs, and our self-doubt, which all combined, can present our biggest obstacles that prevent us from achieving whatever it is in life that we want to achieve.

We can all choose to have that victim mindset, and give explanations and justifications to stay where we are. We can get stuck in a rut, we can make more excuses than answer why we can't do things, but ultimately, the only person that can, or will, change anything about ourselves or our lives is us.

None of us are promised tomorrow, so we need to live our best for today. We need to do what makes us happy—travel, buy the car we've always wanted, or change our job if it depresses us. Life is too short to be depressed or unhappy. Only a select few of us get second chances at life; most of us don't come back.

I enjoy my life but I don't live everyday like it's my last, because if I did that, then I'd either be in jail or dead! I have learned to love life more, especially lately; I think having clarity in my life and sharing it with someone amazing that enjoys challenges as much as I do has made a huge difference. I am more comfortable in myself these days, even when life gets tough. Financially, this is the toughest time it has ever been for mum, myself, and even Amelia. But on the bright side, it's the happiest I've ever been.

We have struggled for so long in every aspect of our lives and we have hit rock bottom more than once, but amazingly, it has bought us all closer together instead of dividing us. As hard as it has gotten at times, we work through these life challenges together and I am grateful for that.

It can be very hard when there is nobody to lean on in tough times.

There are a lot of people in that type of situation, so everyone needs to keep being motivated and excited about their life.

They need to set achievable goals that will push their life forward, get them out from their rock-bottom state through setting small achievable goals, being grateful, and appreciating what they have.

These are the key most important tools for people to have in order to make positive changes in their life.

Amelia and I want to start a family sometime soon; that's my new motivation. I don't want to be a dad who just sits on the sidelines.

Over a year ago, I was at the park with my stepbrother Andrew and his son Tylar. Andrew was on the phone and Tylar wanted to get his kite in the air but he didn't know how to, so he asked me to show him. The reality hit me hard when I wasn't able to run with Tylar to get enough speed to launch the kite into the air. It made me think about my future and having this same moment with my kid.

It's the simple pleasures we take for granted the most, but instead of getting upset about that moment, I now use that day with Tylar in the park as motivation. I see dads and mums walking down the street with a pram or with a child in their arms and I want to do that. The only way I'll make that happen is by fixing myself now. I want to be able to walk with my wife and kids down the street.

So now I use the treadmill every day at the gym, and for more practice, I walk non-stop around the oval on the grass with the dogs on the lead next to Amelia. Incorporating both of those walking exercises into my daily training really helps in correcting my balance and increasing my endurance.

The spasms that I get through my arms, legs, core, and back are pretty severe. For those who don't understand spasms, for someone with a cord injury they are like massive cramps. Sometimes the muscles lock up. Sometimes they shake, and at times it can be very severe. My spasms are one massive hurdle that I'm still trying to push through and overcome. Since the beginning of my recovery, I have incorporated breathing techniques to try and breathe out the contractions and relax my body. Lately, I have made it my routine that as soon as I get out of bed that I do 15 to 20 minutes yoga-style exercises to lengthen my muscles and to warm my body up. I've noticed that after a few weeks, I was able to control the spasms a little easier.

I don't want to get to my last day and realize that there were things I didn't get to experience or wish I should have done or goals I didn't achieve; I've been in that space before. When I was lying on the side of the road seconds after my accident, reality was right in my face, making all those, "I wish I had" statements:

"I wish I had done this…"

"I wish I was a better person to my friends and my family."

"I wish I got to do the snow trips I only dreamed of and talked about."

And the big question: "Is this it? Is this where my journey ends?"

I was lucky enough to have lived a pretty damn full life before my accident. I have travelled the globe more than most adults have. I had a great upbringing; mum and dad always supported me with my sports, whether it was racing BMX, riding motocross, or my snowboarding; they always encouraged me to chase my dreams.

I did a lot of travelling with mum and dad when they were together, then mum and I had our adventures in Switzerland and Bali. I was given many options in my life, but I had to work for them; they weren't handed to me on a silver platter and I didn't expect them to be either. Don't get me wrong, I was a little shit at times, but I look back on my childhood now and I am so grateful for all the opportunities I was given.

I was very grateful for everything that my parents did for me, but I wasn't content with just that; I had so much more that I wanted to do with my life. Life is much harder now, but I was given a second chance. I was one of those select few who get a second shot at life.

That 18-year-old boy who I was did die that day back in June 2000 in a way. I was never the same afterwards—maybe to look at when I was sitting down—but physically and mentally, I was never the same.

Through sheer determination and love, I was given a second chance at life. I was "twice born" and I knew it! I embraced that second chance with a relentless and Never-Give-Up attitude with everything I had and I reminded myself of that every day, After all, I had a lot to be grateful for.

Aside from my injury, I had "twice born" tattooed across my chest. I see it everyday. It is a constant written reminder for me.

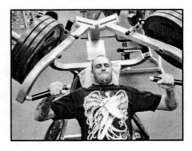

It has been a tough and very hard journey to say the least, but I have no regrets. It has made me the person I am today, especially in the last few years. The only regrets to be had from my accident are what it did to the boys, my family, and my other mates that day and all the emotions they had to deal with. The shock of my accident and the fear and not knowing if I was going to live at that point was obviously very hard for all of them to deal with in those frightening moments on the mountain.

I can't change the past—no one can—but I can learn from it. I used that pain to show everyone around me that I'll be okay. I'll be different, but I'll be happy. Maybe even better than before.

I live a life of physical pain and challenges every day. I've been thrown more hurdles to get over in my life than most people would ever experience in their entire lifetime. Somehow, I'm still standing and still swinging. I could focus on all the bad, but what would that prove? Who would that help? Instead, I focus on what I have and what I can get back. It can always get worse, so I make sure that I appreciate everything I have in my life.

People constantly ask me, "But how did you do it? What's your secret? What did you do differently?"

Amelia gets asked the same thing about her fitness and motivation and how she has the body she has. Her answer is the same as mine: it's all about hard work, diet and healthy eating, determination, and dedication to change and achieve something better. It's about having the will to never give up on your goals and dreams. It's no secret. Too many people want the easy pill the quick fix, but in reality where we live, that's not available.

The only way we can do it is to keep it simple. I trained, I looked after myself, and I learned new skills. I fought every single day and I still do. Sure it got difficult. Sometimes it got really difficult, almost to the point of complete breakdown, but something inside me kept pushing. Something inside me knew I wasn't finished with my story, and that there was so much more to give, to do, to say and to share with people. A few times, I nearly threw it all away from pushing the boundaries too far, but somehow I learned from it and came back stronger and with better knowledge. I'm still learning every day.

Imagine if I listened to the doctors and not to my mum and I just gave up. I wouldn't have my wife, my dogs, or my true understanding of real mates. I wouldn't have the friendship I have with my mum and family or know what true happiness really is. I wouldn't have the belief that I could achieve the impossible.

Only a few weeks before my accident, I was at the gym with Dutchy. As we trained, we noticed a guy in a wheelchair training really hard on the weights.

I turned to Dutchy and said, "Dude, if I was going to be in a wheelchair, I would want to die. That guy has some heart to keep motivated!"

If only I knew what was going to happen to me in just a short time after that day and what challenges I had ahead of me.

Even now, it's the small things I notice.

A few months ago, I was on a spin bike at the gym. As I rode, Amelia sent me a text message. I replied to her text and I looked down and realized my legs had stopped pedaling. I never knew how much I used my concentration to move my legs, until that day. So from then on, whenever I was on the spin bike, I made sure I played games on my phone while pedaling to teach my brain and body to work as one and to multi-task. Now when I go on the treadmill, I look around and try not to focus on looking at my feet all the time. It's a bit hard to text on the treadmill because I'm still not able to walk on the treadmill without holding onto the sidebars. The difficulty is because I move around so much on the equipment, that it's hard to look at the screen. But, I still think outside the box and discover new things and new ways of doing what I used to find so easy to do before my accident.

When I was in hospital, one of the first things they told me was whatever I got back in the first three years was pretty much it; after that, I wouldn't gain much more. I've proved that's bullshit and so have many others.

Compared to when I was first injured to where I am now, I see more and more people getting function and movement back. I guess there are more fighters than ever before. The more one of us fights, the more the next unfortunate injured person will know that there is a chance of recovery even after they've been handed a similar sentence to me. And I say "sentence" because it feels felt like a life sentence when I first had this injury. It has been a very tough, long, unforgiving road, but life was never meant to be easy, and that's the case even if they aren't struck down with a spinal cord injury.

People relate my story to their own life in more ways than one, whether it's goal setting for their company and how to better it, better their staff, their focus, or even to better their personal relationship they are in and to appreciate what they have. Life isn't meant to be boring, so what's the point in being unhappy?

One other reason why I kept my story and recovery to myself for the first 10 years after my accident was for this exact reason: lately, my mum and I have had a select few emails from family members and people with spinal cord injury questioning my recovery, my therapy, and even the extent of my injury.

From day one, I never knew what was going to work, but we decided to go the alternative route as the foundation for my recovery, because the practitioners, the healers and the techniques they used and they way worked on me gave me more hope. When I visit people in hospital and speak with them and their family members, I tell them my story and what we did, and I always make sure I remind them that just because the alternative approach worked for me, it doesn't mean that it will work for them.

Whichever recovery path we choose to take, the result will be different for each person. We can't time it either. Just because I walked within the first year, it doesn't mean that the next person will. Hell, they may even walk quicker than I did, or they may never walk again. Who knows? We cannot compare our injury and recovery to the next person. Spinal cord injury is not black and white; it's a massive grey area!

I always tell people the difference is that they have to be willing to fail more than succeed and know how to handle failure! Hell, I've tried walking on a treadmill since my accident and it has never clicked until now. That has been 13 long hard years.

I have tried more things and failed at more things than I could wish for, but I never regret any of it. It has all come at a huge cost financially and emotionally, but can we really put a price on independence?

I have put myself out there into the world to not only inspire cord injured people, but to inspire everyone. It has taken 13 years for me to say that—I know I can inspire people. In the past, I thought that sounded arrogant, but now I don't think it does. I follow so many people that inspire me on a daily basis and they don't even know that they do—whether it's fitness, work ethics, relationship, business decisions, or any other aspect of life.

We can all get motivation from anywhere. I remember a few months before I had my accident, a motor cross/FMX rider named Carey Hart, did the impossible and back flipped his dirt bike, and he was the first in the world to do so. I was lucky enough to meet him not long after he did it only a short time before my accident. What he did on that bike motivated me in my dark days while in my hospital bed. I watched his video over and over again as motivation to see the impossible be possible.

Sometimes I feel like going back to my old ways of keeping to myself and not having to worry about other people, but that wouldn't be right. I never had someone in my life that truly understood what I went through mentally and physically every day with this injury. The only person that did understand on every level was Bronte, and he isn't here with us anymore. I'll never get him back, but he inspired me to never give up and to try to help as many people as possible.

Life doesn't have to be a lonely existence. A lot of the time, I feel done with having to justify myself and explain my recovery to people. I get over having the feeling that I need to prove "how bad I really was" and still am. I have just learned how to hide it every day. I have enough on my plate, whether it's trying to figure out how to live off very little dollars and be able to afford everyday items like petrol, food, clothes, and pay my bills, and everything else we go through every single day. I could focus on that, but I choose not to. Instead, I focus on my wife, my dogs, my mates, my family, and my health; all the important things that most people take for granted. What right do I have to complain? I'm sure there are a few people in the world who would love to have my problems because theirs are worse.

The moral of my story is this: if we play the victim role, complain, and get upset about how hard we have it, and just stay in that space, keep on doing the same thing over and over and keep on saying the same shit over and over, then we only have ourselves to blame if nothing changes. Life can be bloody hard at the best of times, but it can always get worse, so we need to be grateful for what we have, and fight for our dreams, whether it's physically, emotionally, or even financially.

Unfortunately, there are some instances with certain people that I feel the need to have to carry the MRI of my injured cord to show them how bad it is, just to prove that yes, I really am and was as bad as I say I was. It's hard for people to realize that because they see me vertical and walking; at face value I present that I'm not too bad, but clinically and internally, I still have all the same problems as any other cord injured person; I just don't focus on it.

What I focus on and say to all the doubters who question the extent of my injury and others just like me is:

- There are always options.
- There are alternatives.
- There are many different answers.
- This does not have to be the only answer just because a guy in a white coat says so.
- There is substantial proof in my story alone that went way ahead from what was first said to me in the hospital that it was not possible. There are more people now proving to doctors everyday what is possible, whether it's a cord injury, cancer, brain trauma, or even everyday problems we all face.

I wasn't the brightest kid academically on paper. When I was at school, sometimes I didn't think I would amount to much because I was given an exam score that reflected the exact opposite of what I thought was right. We are all different so how can we all be judged in the same way?

I was the boy who loved looking out the window at school. There was an entire world out there to be discovered and I felt like I was wasting my life at school. But in saying that, I'm glad I graduated. It gave me a sense of relief and that I had accomplished something, even though I didn't think school would help me at the time.

I once saw a little cartoon picture that had this verse written underneath it: "Everybody is a genius but if you judge a fish by its ability to climb a tree, it will live its whole life believing that it is stupid." That is so true in so many ways.

This injury has given me the strength to deal with so many other things on so many levels, like relationship breakups, financial problems, not always being able to go to the places I would like to go to and do things I would normally like to do. In my eyes, all these things are so irrelevant and 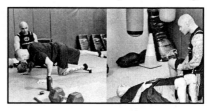 pale in comparison once I've gone through losing the ability to function and losing control of my own life in many areas. To come back from that much loss and pretty much get it all back gives me the most powerful feeling I could ever have of self-gratification. You have to believe in yourself 100 percent and believe that anything is possible.

I try to set a new goal each week that will help to improve myself in one way or another, whether it's to set myself up with work in doing my talks, or mentoring someone, physically improving my body and fitness levels, or even better—my relationship with my wife—and to be happy right where I am in life. Every week, I try to achieve something new because if I introduce something new into my life, I get to go beyond my daily limitations and expectations and see what's possible.

"New" is the greatest gift I can give myself because it keeps me from being stagnant and complacent in my life. Like I said before, it pushes me way ahead of what is not possible into everything that is possible.

When I wake up every day and I see those inked words across my chest, "TWICE BORN," I know that I am one of the select few that have been given a second shot. I know that I have been given the greatest gift—I have been given the gift of my life back—and it's a gift that I can share with everyone through being here to tell my story and get the message out that with determination, dedication, work, belief, and Never-Give-Up attitude. Everything is possible!

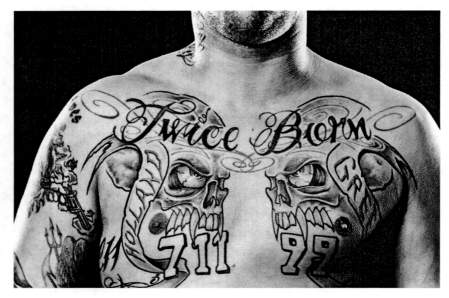

# Glossary of Australian Terminology

## Mate

The one word that most of the World probably associates with Australia is the word mate.

'G'day mate' is a form of greeting that many Australians use. Some use the word mate instead of friend.

A real mate: someone so close to you, someone who no matter what has your back no matter what, someone you can totally rely on, and someone you respect and totally admire.

'Mateship' is a concept that can be traced back to early colonial times. The harsh environment in which convicts and new settlers found themselves meant that men and women closely relied on each other for all sorts of help. In Australia, a 'mate' is more than just a friend. It's a term that implies a sense of shared experience, mutual respect and unconditional assistance. Mateship is a term traditionally used among men, and it is a term frequently used to describe the relationship between men during times of challenge. The popular notion of mateship came to the fore during the First World War. Extract from an article: 'Mateship, Diggers and Wartime' an Australian Government Publication (www.australia.gov.au/about-australia/australian-story/mateship-diggers-and-wartime)

## Whinge

To complain or protest in an annoying or persistent manner; whine.

## Ute/Utility Vehicle

A light truck with an open body and sides. In Josh's case, his SS Ute was a high-powered vehicle with an open rear tray with sides.

## Haunt

Somewhere you frequently hang out, somewhere you enjoy. It could be a restaurant, a club, a hotel, or a pub.

# Josh's Biography

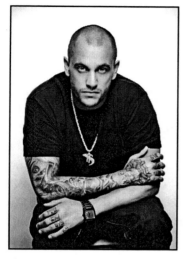

Josh Wood was born in 1981 in Frankston, Melbourne Australia, and from the moment he could move he was active. He rode a mini BMX bike before he could walk and this set him up for a life of action sports. Graduating from high school, he pursued his dream of becoming a professional snowboarder. That dream came to a crashing halt when an aerial snowboard jump went terribly wrong. In a split second, Josh became a quadriplegic. Despite the medical team's prognosis that he would never get out of bed due to the severity of spinal cord damage, he defied the odds, rose up, and through self-healing methods and determination, he was able to walk again. From this point onwards, Josh decided to bring his message to scores of people who face similar challenges, as well as to everyday people from all walks of life. Josh is a published author, motivational speaker, an inspirational advocate for self-healing, and a man with a simple message for the world: Never Give Up!

# Kay's Biography

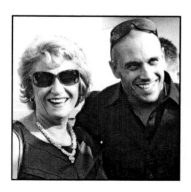

Kay Ledson, Josh Wood's mother, was thrown into the scary world of spinal cord injury when her son had his snowboarding accident. Ledson's background of financial services hardly prepared her for what she had to deal with for her son's catastrophic injury. Thirteen years ago, while the Internet was still in its infancy, Ledson and Wood made the decision not to research spinal cord injury; they decided very quickly that every injury was different, and therefore they approached Wood's rehabilitation and recovery as though he was injured—not disabled. Ledson was a stickler for positive language to be used around her son and how he was to be treated by his medical team. Those first months were a nightmare for Ledson and Wood as they tried to understand this injury and all that came with it. With no one to ask or mentor them, Ledson and Wood relied on friends from Alternative healing modalities to work with them.

Over the years, Ledson and Wood have mentored many families. Ledson worked with Wood in writing his book throughout the years and it has been an amazing experience for her. They are proud to be able to share their experience with the world. Ledson helped Wood and Anton in the writing process by providing an accurate story of Wood's ongoing recovery, especially from her perspective as a supportive and involved mother in the recovery process. Ledson has established Warrior Momz to provide advocacy, mentoring, and advice for families going through the cruel and unrelenting spinal cord injury. Even though Warrior Momz is small in numbers, their outreach is growing worldwide. Ledson and Wood are excited to bring this book to the world for not only those with a spinal cord injury, but also for anyone who dreams and believes that anything is possible.

## Angeleah's Biography

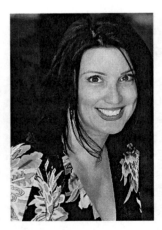

Angeleah Anton started writing stories as soon as she mastered how to hold a pen. She has followed a storyteller's path through her work as an accomplished author, freelance writer, and journalist. She also has experience as a counsellor, Neuro Linguistics Programming Master Practitioner, and motivational speaker. While co-presenting on a spiritual community radio show in Los Angeles, she caught the attention of Josh Wood's mother, Kay Ledson. With the idea of sharing Josh's inspirational healing journey with Angeleah's radio listeners, Kay and Angeleah connected. Soon afterwards, Angeleah met Josh, who gave a detailed first-hand account of his tenacious recovery journey. The decision was made for Angeleah to co-author Josh's book and to help bring his inspirational message to the world.

A self-confessed "social network butterfly," today Angeleah continues to blog and contributes regularly to her social media sites, website, and community forums. She travels between both her home bases of Melbourne, Australia and Los Angeles, USA, for seminars and motivational speaking engagements.

# Information

Josh Wood is an inspirational speaker who spends time travelling between his home base in Melbourne, Australia and Los Angeles, United States, for speaking engagements. He has spoken about his incredible story of beating the odds at financial services conferences, keynote speaking engagements, motivational speaking events, and training workshops.

Josh has also appeared on several radio programs, on television, at schools, and at fundraisers. His story has been covered in several Melbourne newspapers and magazines, such as the Financial Planning Magazine and Extreme Sports Magazine. He has also been featured in the book Chiropractic for the Soul.

**Face Book Sites**
JoshWood
WoodyDitchTheStick

**Website**
www.joshwood.com.au

**Twitter**
@woody_jjw

**LinkedIn**
Josh Wood

**Kay Ledson's Website**
www.LedsonGroupAmerica.com

If you want to get on the path to be a published author by
**Influence Publishing** please go to
**www.InspireABook.com**

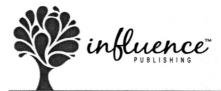

Inspiring books that influence change

More information on our other titles and how to submit
your own proposal can be found at
**www.InfluencePublishing.com**

CPSIA information can be obtained at www.ICGtesting.com
Printed in the USA
LVOW10s0127141013

356689LV00005B/6/P